Annette B. Natow, Ph.D., R.D., and Jo-Ann Heslin, M.A., R.D., are the authors of twenty-four books on nutrition, including *No-Nonsense Nutrition for Your Baby's First Year* and *No-Nonsense Nutrition for Kids*. Both are former faculty members of Adelphi University and the State University of New York, Downstate Medical Center. They are editors of the *Journal of Nutrition for the Elderly* and serve as editorial board members for *Environmental Nutrition Newsletter*. In addition, Heslin is a frequent contributor to *Healthy Kids* and *American Baby*. She had a monthly column in *Childbirth Educator* for five years.

Natow and Heslin have also taught nutrition classes to pregnant parents for more than twenty years and have worked with major food companies to develop public health nutrition programs for pregnant women.

Books by Annette B. Natow and Jo-Ann Heslin

The Antioxidant Vitamin Counter
The Calorie Counter
The Carbohydrate, Fiber, and Sugar Counter
The Cholesterol Counter (Fifth Edition)
Count On a Healthy Pregnancy
The Diabetes Carbohydrate and Calorie Counter
Eating Out Food Counter
The Fat Attack Plan
The Fat Counter (Fourth Edition)
The Food Shopping Counter
Megadoses
The Most Complete Food Counter
No-Nonsense Nutrition for Kids
The Pocket Encyclopedia of Nutrition
The Pocket Fat Counter (Second Edition)
The Pocket Protein Counter
The Pregnancy Nutrition Counter
The Protein Counter
The Sodium Counter
The Supermarket Nutrition Counter (Second Edition)

Published by POCKET BOOKS

For orders other than by individual consumers, Pocket Books grants a discount on the purchase of **10 or more** copies of single titles for special markets or premium use. For further details, please write to the Vice President of Special Markets, Pocket Books, 1230 Avenue of the Americas, 9th Floor, New York, NY 10020-1586.

For information on how individual consumers can place orders, please write to Mail Order Department, Simon & Schuster Inc., 100 Front Street, Riverside, NJ 08075.

COUNT ON A HEALTHY PREGNANCY

Annette B. Natow, Ph.D., R.D.

Jo-Ann Heslin, M.A., R.D.

Illustrations by
Vicki Kalajian Heit

POCKET BOOKS

New York   London   Toronto   Sydney   Tokyo   Singapore

An *Original* Publication of POCKET BOOKS

POCKET BOOKS, a division of Simon & Schuster Inc.
1230 Avenue of the Americas, New York, NY 10020

ISBN: 0-671-02563-5

First Pocket Books printing September 1999

10 9 8 7 6 5 4 3 2 1

POCKET and colophon are registered trademarks of Simon & Schuster Inc.

Cover photo by VCG/FPG International

Text design by Stanley S. Drate/Folio Graphics Co., Inc.

Printed in the U.S.A.

"At no time is a diet . . . going to bring as big a return as when given to the mother upon whom an infant is depending."

Mary Swartz Rose, Ph.D.
Feeding the Family
Macmillan, 1919

To all our babies:
Allen, Laura, Steven, Kristen, Karen,
George, Sara, Emily, Meryl,
and those yet to come.

———————————

A special thanks to all the pregnant women who have asked us questions over the years; to Judith Nolte, Editor in Chief, *American Baby* magazine; to Kathy, Gina, Stephanie, and Ruth, who reviewed the book; to Steven Natow, M.D., and Stephen Llano; and to our editor, Jane Cavolina; and our agent Nancy Trichter.

———————————

"*Count On a Healthy Pregnancy* babies the expectant mother through a nutritionally healthy pregnancy, offering the best odds for a new life."

Ruth Pleva, M.S.W., C.S.W., A.C.C.E.

PLANNING AHEAD

You become a mother at the moment of conception, caring for and feeding your unborn child. Most of us, however, do not find out we are mothers until our first missed period or later, often 4 to 8 weeks into our baby's development. The first 4 to 12 weeks of pregnancy are extremely important, when your baby is forming major organ systems like the spinal cord, heart, and brain.

If you are thinking about pregnancy, think about caring for your unborn baby from here on: eat well, exercise, limit caffeine, and don't use drugs, alcohol, or cigarettes. Then when you get the wonderful news that you are pregnant, you'll be confident that you are already taking good care of your baby.

INTRODUCTION

You may have just found out you're pregnant or you're waiting patiently for the home pregnancy test to give you great news. You're excited and full of expectations, but you're also a little worried about what you've gotten yourself into.

Your partner is great—supportive, excited, caring—but he's never been pregnant, and it's your body that's experiencing all these different and unusual sensations. You can't help wondering if this is normal and if you and your baby are doing okay.

We want to assure you that everything that's happening is normal and you can *count on a healthy pregnancy*. Most pregnancies are healthy, happy experiences. We know that, because we've had children and coached hundreds of women through their pregnancies.

We want to coach you, too. Sharing your experience week by week, letting you know what's happening to you and your growing baby.

Enjoy the next nine months—pregnancy is an experience unmatched by any other. *How are the two of you doing? Just fine!*

PART I

YOUR
HEALTHY
PREGNANCY

GETTING STARTED

Nothing is more exciting than experiencing the week-by-week changes happening during a healthy pregnancy. How you take care of yourself right now directly affects the development of your baby's brain, heart, lungs, and other vital organs. The two of you are an inseparable pair.

Women who eat well throughout pregnancy and gain the appropriate amount of weight are more likely to have healthy babies than women who gain too little or too much. When you eat well, your baby receives needed nutrients, passed from your bloodstream through the bridge between you (the placenta) and into your baby's blood supply. When you eat poorly, skipping meals or making poor food choices, neither of you gets the nutrients needed. You're a team that shares available resources.

Over the next 36 weeks, we'll offer you a lot of nutrition information to keep both of you healthy. But to get started right now, we suggest that you pick one day each week on which to keep a record of everything you eat on the "Pregnancy Food Checklist." Look up the nutrient content of each food in Part II, Food Values, to see if you are reaching the nutrient goals for pregnancy. If not, you can adjust your diet by making different choices.

Every food you eat contains nutrients. Though all nutrients are important, certain key nutrients are especially important during pregnancy—protein, calcium, vitamin C, folic acid (a B vitamin), and iron. We'll discuss all of these with you in more detail as the weeks go by. The foods that are rich sources of key nutrients will provide many other nutrients, too. To be sure you are getting all the key nutrients daily, aim for:

2–3 servings of protein-rich foods
3 servings of calcium-rich foods
5 or more fruits and vegetables
6 or more servings of breads, grains, and cereals

PREGNANCY TESTS

These tests provide a great deal of information and help your health care practitioner see into the future. Many of these tests are done only once, and some may not be needed.

Pregnancy test. A blood test to confirm your pregnancy.

Blood pressure. Taken regularly to monitor the small changes expected during pregnancy. Your health care practitioner is watching for sudden increases, which need to be handled right away.

Blood and Rh tests. Blood tests that tell your blood type (A, B, AB, or O) and Rh status (positive or negative). Rh factor is a protein you may or may not have in your blood cells.

STDs. Sexually transmitted diseases like chlamydia, syphilis, gonorrhea, and AIDS can be passed to your baby. If detected and treated early, the illnesses can be minimized.

Urine tests. Monitors for protein, blood, bacteria, or sugar that may signal a problem that needs attention.

Ultrasound. Also called a sonogram, this test can tell the size of a baby, the due date, the progress of growth, the presence of more than one baby, or the cause of problems. A wand is passed over your belly, emitting sound waves that produce a picture of your baby on a TV monitor.

Chorionic villus sampling (CVS). A test that may be done between week 10 and week 12, which can detect genetic problems.

Hepatitis B virus (HBV) screening. A blood test for HBV, which can be transmitted to your baby at birth.

Alpha-fetoprotein (AFT). A protein found in amniotic fluid. A higher-than-usual or lower-than-usual level may detect a possible problem.

Amniocentesis. Usually done between week 15 and week 18 of pregnancy to tell the sex of your baby and help to detect problems.

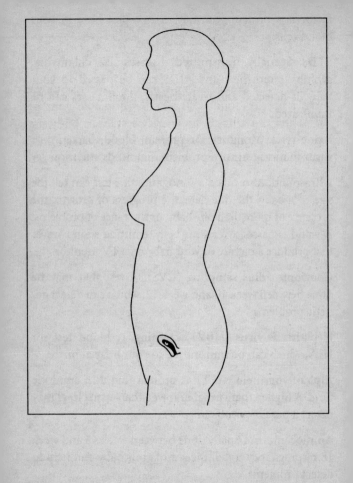

WEEK 4

You've been pregnant for almost a month, but you may have just found out when you missed your period and did a home pregnancy test. Your body may be giving you signals that something is up. It's time to make an appointment with your health care practitioner.

FIRST SIGNS OF PREGNANCY

Missing a period
Tender breasts
Feeling very tired and sleepy
Being very sensitive to odors
Metallic taste in your mouth
Slight rise in body temperature—about one degree
More vaginal discharge than normal
Need to use the bathroom often

HOW ARE THE TWO OF YOU DOING?

Your baby is very tiny, about the size of a letter "o" on this page.

You haven't gained any weight, and no one, except those you tell, will know that you are pregnant. But a great many things are happening. Your baby is growing and changing every day.

All this growth and development, especially now when your baby's organs and body structures are forming, is supported by you and the foods you eat.

Each day aim for:

2–3 servings of protein-rich foods

3 servings of calcium-rich foods

5 or more fruits and vegetables

6 or more servings of breads, grains, and cereals

Do I really have to eat all those servings every day?

Serving sizes you get at a restaurant or even those you serve yourself at home may be far larger than an "average" serving size. The visual cues on the opposite page will help you estimate "average" portions.

Now you can see that it is easier than you realized to eat all those servings each day. A plateful of spaghetti always equals more than one serving. A side salad could easily equal two servings. And an average glass of milk is likely to contain 10 to 12 ounces, more than an average serving size. The servings you should aim for each day are not as large as you imagined, and they are definitely needed to ensure that you and your baby get all the key nutrients.

1 CUP MEASURE
(equals 8 ounces,
or 1 serving)

1 serving milk, yogurt, cooked
pasta, dry cereal, fresh salad

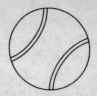

TENNIS BALL
(equals 1/2 cup,
or 1 medium fruit)

1/2 cup cooked vegetable,
fruit salad, canned fruit,
mashed potatoes, cooked rice,
cooked beans, cooked cereal;
1 medium apple, peach,
tomato, orange

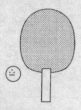

PING-PONG BALL
(equals 1 ounce,
or 2 tablespoons)

1 ounce cheese; 2 tablespoons
salad dressing, gravy, peanut
butter, cream cheese,
guacamole, sour cream,
mayonnaise

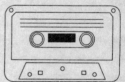

TAPE CASSETTE
(equals 4 ounces of boneless
meat, fish, or poultry)

4-ounce fillet of fish,
4-ounce hamburger,
4-ounce boneless steak,
1/2 chicken breast,
1 center cut pork chop

WEEK 4

PREGNANCY FOOD CHECKLIST

Goals:
- 2–3 servings of protein-rich foods
- 3 servings of calcium-rich foods
- 5 or more fruits and vegetables
- 6 or more servings of breads, grains, and cereals

	Calories	Protein	Vit C	Folic Acid	Calcium	Iron
Breakfast						
Subtotal	___	___	___	___	___	___
Snack						
Subtotal	___	___	___	___	___	___
Lunch						
Subtotal	___	___	___	___	___	___
Snack						
Subtotal	___	___	___	___	___	___
Dinner						
Subtotal	___	___	___	___	___	___
Snack						
Subtotal	___	___	___	___	___	___
Daily total	___	___	___	___	___	___
Daily Nutrient Goals	2200	60	70	300–400*	1000	10–15**

* You need 600 mcg of folic acid daily, but some of that comes from your prenatal supplement.

** You need 30 mg of iron daily, but some of that comes from your prenatal supplement.

WEEK 4

Appointments:

Date _____ Time _____

Date _____ Time _____

Remember to find out if _____

_____

_____

Goals:

Next week I will _____

_____

My weight is _____

Your baby's growth is continuous, requiring a steady supply of nutrients. If you skip a meal, ask yourself, "Who's feeding my baby?"

WEEK 5

HOW ARE THE TWO OF YOU DOING?

Your baby hasn't grown much larger, but his central nervous system, heart, muscular structure, and bones are in their early stages.

You haven't changed much either, but your body is definitely signaling you that something is going on.

YOUR DUE DATE

Pregnancy lasts about 280 days, or 40 weeks. To estimate your due date, add 7 days to the date of your last period and subtract 3 months. Only 1 woman out of 20 actually has her baby on her due date; 90% deliver the week before or the week after.

My due date is _____

Why is folic acid so important in pregnancy?

Folic acid, a B vitamin, helps to form red and white blood cells and the correct genetic material inside every cell in the body. Since your baby is making billions of cells during the next nine months, it's obvious why this vitamin is so important. In addition, research has shown that adequate folic acid can prevent serious birth defects and may help prevent heart disease.

Your prenatal vitamins contain folic acid. It is important to take them every day. Food sources of folic acid will add to your daily total.

Because this vitamin is so important, and because it is estimated that only one-third of women get enough of it daily, the Food and Drug Administration requires all enriched breads, cereals, and pastas to be fortified with folic acid. Ready-to-eat cereal is an excellent source. Other good sources are:

asparagus	peas
Brussels sprouts	wheat germ
broccoli	enriched bread
collard greens	enriched pasta
romaine lettuce	white flour
spinach	ready-to-eat cereals
turnip greens	pinto beans
orange juice	lima beans
oranges	lentils
cashews	peanuts

Aim for 300 to 400 micrograms of folic acid from food choices each day. You may not always meet your goal, but make every effort to select foods rich in this important nutrient.

WEEK 5

PREGNANCY FOOD CHECKLIST

Goals:
- 2–3 servings of protein-rich foods
- 3 servings of calcium-rich foods
- 5 or more fruits and vegetables
- 6 or more servings of breads, grains, and cereals

	Calories	Protein	Vit C	Folic Acid	Calcium	Iron
Breakfast						
Subtotal	____	____	____	____	____	____
Snack						
Subtotal	____	____	____	____	____	____
Lunch						
Subtotal	____	____	____	____	____	____
Snack						
Subtotal	____	____	____	____	____	____
Dinner						
Subtotal	____	____	____	____	____	____
Snack						
Subtotal	____	____	____	____	____	____
Daily total	____	____	____	____	____	____
Daily Nutrient Goals	2200	60	70	300–400*	1000	10–15**

* You need 600 mcg of folic acid daily, but some of that comes from your prenatal supplement.

** You need 30 mg of iron daily, but some of that comes from your prenatal supplement.

WEEK 5

Appointments:

Date _____ Time _____

Date _____ Time _____

Remember to find out if _____

_____

_____

Goals:

Next week I will _____

_____

❀

Smoking isn't good for either of you. It interferes with the use of the key nutrients vitamin C and folic acid. Expectant mothers who smoke are more likely to have pregnancy complications. Their babies are often smaller at birth, and new research suggests that babies exposed to nicotine before birth may be more likely to smoke when they get older.

❀

WEEK 6

HOW ARE THE TWO OF YOU DOING?

Your baby's body is taking shape; the head is now obvious. The brain and eyes are forming, and her heart has begun to beat. Tiny limb buds can be seen, which will grow into arms and legs.

You may have gained a few pounds, or perhaps you've lost a few if you've been nauseated. Your clothes may feel slightly tight around the waist, and your breasts are getting bigger.

Uterus: The sac holding your baby. It expands and stretches to accommodate your growing baby.

Placenta: The bridge between the two of you extending from the wall of the uterus to your baby. It's used to deliver nutrients to the baby and carry wastes away from her.

Amniotic fluid: The clear fluid in which your baby floats.

I'm so nauseous! Will this go on for nine months?

Pregnancy nausea, with or without vomiting, is usually called morning sickness, though it can occur at any time during the day. Almost half of all pregnant women experience morning sickness beginning around the 6th week. The good news is that it usually gets better or goes away by the end of the 12th week.

You can do a number of things to make yourself feel better. Many women experience a wave a nausea when they jump out of bed in the morning, and this may set the stage for discomfort all day. So don't jump out of bed. Set the alarm a few minutes early. Wake up, but don't get up. Leave a few crackers next to the bed each night. Stay in bed in the morning and munch on them, even though you may not feel like eating. Don't worry about crumbs. Now get up slowly and start your day. For many this is enough to solve the whole morning-sickness problem.

Vomiting, other than in the morning, is rare, but queasiness can creep up on you at any time during the day. Eating often helps. Bread, cereal, unbuttered popcorn, toast, or a baked potato will go down nicely and will calm your stomach. Many women also report that it helps to sip cold beverages rather than drink them. Ginger has anti-nausea properties, and many women find sipping cold ginger ale helps. Don't use herbal supplements without checking with your health care practitioner.

Some women find that certain smells, like brewing coffee, can trigger nausea. If smells bother you, try to avoid them.

Though morning sickness is no fun, those women who are bothered with it, statistically, have fewer complications later on.

WEEK 6

PREGNANCY FOOD CHECKLIST

Goals:
- 2–3 servings of protein-rich foods
- 3 servings of calcium-rich foods
- 5 or more fruits and vegetables
- 6 or more servings of breads, grains, and cereals

	Calories	Protein	Vit C	Folic Acid	Calcium	Iron
Breakfast						
Subtotal	____	____	____	____	____	____
Snack						
Subtotal	____	____	____	____	____	____
Lunch						
Subtotal	____	____	____	____	____	____
Snack						
Subtotal	____	____	____	____	____	____
Dinner						
Subtotal	____	____	____	____	____	____
Snack						
Subtotal	____	____	____	____	____	____
Daily total	____	____	____	____	____	____
Daily Nutrient Goals	2200	60	70	300–400*	1000	10–15**

* You need 600 mcg of folic acid daily, but some of that comes from your prenatal supplement.
** You need 30 mg of iron daily, but some of that comes from your prenatal supplement.

WEEK 6

Appointments:

Date _____ Time _____

Date _____ Time _____

Remember to find out if _____

_____

_____

Goals:

Next week I will _____

_____

❋

You will spend a good deal of the beginning and end of
your pregnancy in the bathroom. Location is everything,
and your bladder, unfortunately, is located between your
enlarging uterus and your pubic bone, reducing its capac-
ity and giving you the urge to go every 10 minutes. This
annoyance will pass shortly, only to return just before delivery when your baby's head drops down and presses on
your bladder once again. Don't stop drinking fluids; it
won't help.

❋

WEEK 7

HOW ARE THE TWO OF YOU DOING?

Your baby, your own little sweet pea, is about the size of a green pea. His arms have gotten longer and his hands are beginning to form.

You should be seeing a little weight gain by now, and although you cannot feel it, your baby has begun to move around.

An **embryo** is a baby in the first 8 weeks of pregnancy, when major organ systems are forming.

A **fetus** is the developing baby during the rest of the pregnancy.

I eat mostly vegetarian meals. Will I get enough protein for my baby to grow?

Meat, fish, and poultry are the most obvious protein-rich foods, but you get some protein from most foods you eat. Plant protein sources include cereals, peas, dried beans, nuts, seeds, peanut butter, and tofu—all of which are excellent sources. And don't forget milk, eggs, and cheese. Most people eat twice the protein they need each day, so there is no need to worry about your vegetarian choices.

Protein-rich foods provide the building material needed to produce the billions of tiny cells that transform your baby from a microscopic embryo to a healthy full-term baby. And you're growing too—breast tissue, uterine tissue, the placenta, and new blood cells. All this maintenance, building, and repair requires extra protein—2 to 3 servings a day.

WEEK 7

PREGNANCY FOOD CHECKLIST

Goals:
- 2–3 servings of protein-rich foods
- 3 servings of calcium-rich foods
- 5 or more fruits and vegetables
- 6 or more servings of breads, grains, and cereals

	Calories	Protein	Vit C	Folic Acid	Calcium	Iron
Breakfast						
Subtotal	___	___	___	___	___	___
Snack						
Subtotal	___	___	___	___	___	___
Lunch						
Subtotal	___	___	___	___	___	___
Snack						
Subtotal	___	___	___	___	___	___
Dinner						
Subtotal	___	___	___	___	___	___
Snack						
Subtotal	___	___	___	___	___	___
Daily total	___	___	___	___	___	___
Daily Nutrient Goals	2200	60	70	300–400*	1000	10–15**

* You need 600 mcg of folic acid daily, but some of that comes from your prenatal supplement.

** You need 30 mg of iron daily, but some of that comes from your prenatal supplement.

WEEK 7

Appointments:

Date _____ Time _____

Date _____ Time _____

Remember to find out if _____

_____

_____

Goals:

Next week I will _____

_____

❀

You should not eat raw meat dishes such as beef carpaccio and steak tartare while you are pregnant. Also avoid raw fish, including sushi and seviche, and say no to raw and soft-cooked eggs, game, sport fish, and foods that are cooked rare. These foods may carry bacteria, contaminants, or heavy metals that might be harmful to you or your developing baby.

❀

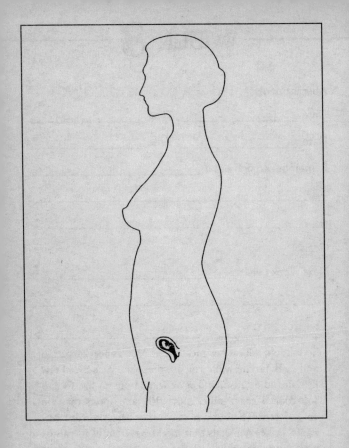

WEEK 8

HOW ARE THE TWO OF YOU DOING?

Your baby is the size of a pinto bean. Eyelid folds are forming. The tip of the nose and ears can be seen. His arms are longer, and he has elbows.

You may feel some tightening or mild cramping in your lower abdomen or sides as your uterus stretches and grows. As long as these are pesky but not sharp pains, there's nothing to worry about. Your uterus is about the size of a grapefruit, causing your stomach to protrude slightly.

I'm so thirsty. Is that normal?

Doctors have known for decades that a moderate water accumulation during pregnancy is a strong indicator of your baby's proper growth. Some women gain as much as 11 pounds of fluid, plus 4 cups of amniotic fluid, plus a quart and a half of extra blood during pregnancy. No wonder you're thirsty!

To meet this extra fluid need you'll need ten 8-ounce glasses of liquid a day. Two to 4 cups of water come from the foods you eat, like soups, fruits, and vegetables that are high in water. The rest should come from beverages—tap water, bottled water, mineral water, milk, fruit juice, fruit punch, fruit nectar, lemonade, and seltzer are all good choices.

WEEK 8

PREGNANCY FOOD CHECKLIST

Goals:
- 2–3 servings of protein-rich foods
- 3 servings of calcium-rich foods
- 5 or more fruits and vegetables
- 6 or more servings of breads, grains, and cereals

	Calories	Protein	Vit C	Folic Acid	Calcium	Iron
Breakfast						
Subtotal	___	___	___	___	___	___
Snack						
Subtotal	___	___	___	___	___	___
Lunch						
Subtotal	___	___	___	___	___	___
Snack						
Subtotal	___	___	___	___	___	___
Dinner						
Subtotal	___	___	___	___	___	___
Snack						
Subtotal	___	___	___	___	___	___
Daily total	___	___	___	___	___	___
Daily Nutrient Goals	2200	60	70	300–400*	1000	10–15**

* You need 600 mcg of folic acid daily, but some of that comes from your prenatal supplement.
** You need 30 mg of iron daily, but some of that comes from your prenatal supplement.

WEEK 8

Appointments:

Date _____ Time _____

Date _____ Time _____

Remember to find out if _____

_____

_____

Goals:

Next week I will _____

_____

My weight is _____

It's unlike you to cry during a sad movie. And taking a nap—you, the human dynamo who could live on 4 hours of sleep. What's going on? The hormonal changes of early pregnancy are responsible for these developments as well as for the changes, both good and bad, in your hair texture and complexion. Everything is normal!

WEEK 9

HOW ARE THE TWO OF YOU DOING?

Your baby is the size of a green olive and is beginning to look like a miniature human.

You are seeing your waistline getting thicker as your weight slowly creeps up.

How much weight should I gain during pregnancy?

Your weight gain is an important way to monitor the well-being of your developing baby. Research has shown that women who gain between 26 and 35 pounds have the healthiest babies. You'll hardly notice your weight gain in the first 3 months of pregnancy. During the middle of pregnancy your weight gain is slow, steady, and obvious. In the last 3 months, you could easily gain a pound a week, as your baby goes through her last growth spurt before birth.

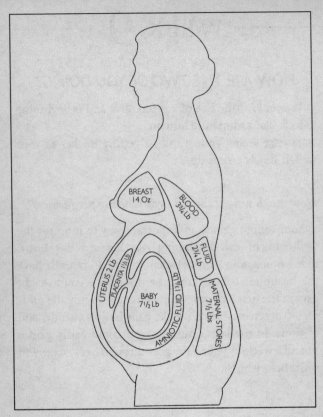

PREGNANCY WEIGHT GAIN

WEEK 9

PREGNANCY FOOD CHECKLIST

Goals:
- 2–3 servings of protein-rich foods
- 3 servings of calcium-rich foods
- 5 or more fruits and vegetables
- 6 or more servings of breads, grains, and cereals

	Calories	Protein	Vit C	Folic Acid	Calcium	Iron
Breakfast						
Subtotal	____	____	____	____	____	____
Snack						
Subtotal	____	____	____	____	____	____
Lunch						
Subtotal	____	____	____	____	____	____
Snack						
Subtotal	____	____	____	____	____	____
Dinner						
Subtotal	____	____	____	____	____	____
Snack						
Subtotal	____	____	____	____	____	____
Daily total	____	____	____	____	____	____
Daily Nutrient Goals	2200	60	70	300–400*	1000	10–15**

* You need 600 mcg of folic acid daily, but some of that comes from your prenatal supplement.

** You need 30 mg of iron daily, but some of that comes from your prenatal supplement.

WEEK 9

Appointments:

Date _____ Time _____

Date _____ Time _____

Remember to find out if _____

_____ _____

_____

Goals:

Next week I will _____

_____

Every pregnant woman wants a healthy baby. It might help you worry less to know that major birth defects happen in only 3% of all pregnancies. Most babies arrive perfect and beautiful, too!

WEEK 10

HOW ARE THE TWO OF YOU DOING?

Your baby is about the size of a small plum.

You are starting to think about buying maternity clothes. You're experiencing many changes in your body and learning to cope with being pregnant. You wonder if your partner still finds you attractive. (Many men think pregnant women are beautiful.) You're feeling very emotional and somewhat vulnerable. This is the time to pamper yourself a little, take care of yourself. Talk about your concerns with your partner, with your health care practitioner, and with friends who have been pregnant. You'll be pleasantly surprised to find out that what you are feeling is normal.

My mother told me to drink at least 4 glasses of milk a day. Do I really need that much?

You should aim for 3 servings of calcium-rich foods each day. They don't all have to be milk. Yogurt, frozen yogurt, and cheese are other excellent sources, as is calcium-fortified orange juice, which is also high in vitamin C, another key nutrient. Stick with lowfat cheese, nonfat yogurt, and lowfat or fat-free milk, all of which have as much calcium as the regular varieties, or even more, with much less fat.

If you have a stomachache, bloating, gas, or diarrhea shortly after drinking milk, you may be lactose intolerant—unable to digest the milk sugar lactose. Try instead low-lactose milk, chocolate milk, pudding, custard, hard cheese, yogurt, kefir, or buttermilk—all may be better tolerated. Or you can rely on nondairy calcium sources like canned sardines and salmon with bones, calcium-fortified orange juice, broccoli, tofu, spinach, and other greens. Most experts feel that a pregnant woman should try to get at least half of her daily calcium from food because calcium-rich foods are excellent sources of other needed nutrients. When necessary, the rest can be provided as a supplement. Your health care practitioner can help you with this.

WEEK 10

PREGNANCY FOOD CHECKLIST

Goals:
- 2–3 servings of protein-rich foods
- 3 servings of calcium-rich foods
- 5 or more fruits and vegetables
- 6 or more servings of breads, grains, and cereals

	Calories	Protein	Vit C	Folic Acid	Calcium	Iron
Breakfast						
Subtotal	____	____	____	____	____	____
Snack						
Subtotal	____	____	____	____	____	____
Lunch						
Subtotal	____	____	____	____	____	____
Snack						
Subtotal	____	____	____	____	____	____
Dinner						
Subtotal	____	____	____	____	____	____
Snack						
Subtotal	____	____	____	____	____	____
Daily total	____	____	____	____	____	____
Daily Nutrient Goals	2200	60	70	300–400*	1000	10–15**

* You need 600 mcg of folic acid daily, but some of that comes from your prenatal supplement.

** You need 30 mg of iron daily, but some of that comes from your prenatal supplement.

WEEK 10

Appointments:

Date _____ Time _____

Date _____ Time _____

Remember to find out if _____

_____

_____

Goals:

Next week I will _____

_____

❋

Raw milk, cheese made from unpasteurized milk, and unpasteurized juice like seasonal apple cider may contain
bacteria that could make you sick and be harmful to your
developing baby.

❋

WEEK 11

HOW ARE THE TWO OF YOU DOING?

Your baby looks like a small person with a very large head. He even has fingernails on his tiny hands.

You are nearing the end of your first trimester and beginning to "look" pregnant.

TRIMESTERS

First: Months 1, 2, and 3, the time from conception through the development of your baby's vital organs.

Second: Months 4, 5, and 6, the middle of pregnancy. Your baby is completely formed, but refinement of organs and body systems happens.

Third: Months 7, 8, and 9, the home stretch as your baby goes through the final growth spurt before birth, tripling her weight and growing in length.

My friend was anemic when she was pregnant. How can I avoid that?

Many women are anemic during pregnancy. You can avoid this by taking your prenatal vitamin supplement and adding iron-rich foods to your daily meals. Many protein-rich foods—meat, eggs, and beans—are also rich in iron. Other good sources are

baked beans	peanuts
blueberries	peas
chickpeas	poultry
enriched bread and cereal	prune juice
fish	raisins
lima beans	spinach

Your need for iron doubles during pregnancy. Getting enough from food alone can be a real challenge. We'd recommend you try to get at least 10 to 15 milligrams of iron a day from food, with the rest from an iron supplement. Many things help or hinder the absorption of iron. Meals containing meat or a source of vitamin C, like tomatoes or orange juice, help. Whole grains, soy, and tea reduce absorption.

Some refer to iron as the body's gold—needed in very small amounts but precious. Your baby needs iron to produce his new blood supply and to lay down some iron stores to be used in the first months of life. You need extra iron because your blood volume has increased. Make a special effort to include this key nutrient daily.

WEEK 11

PREGNANCY FOOD CHECKLIST

Goals:
- 2–3 servings of protein-rich foods
- 3 servings of calcium-rich foods
- 5 or more fruits and vegetables
- 6 or more servings of breads, grains, and cereals

	Calories	Protein	Vit C	Folic Acid	Calcium	Iron
Breakfast						
Subtotal	___	___	___	___	___	___
Snack						
Subtotal	___	___	___	___	___	___
Lunch						
Subtotal	___	___	___	___	___	___
Snack						
Subtotal	___	___	___	___	___	___
Dinner						
Subtotal	___	___	___	___	___	___
Snack						
Subtotal	___	___	___	___	___	___
Daily total	___	___	___	___	___	___
Daily Nutrient Goals	2200	60	70	300–400*	1000	10–15**

* You need 600 mcg of folic acid daily, but some of that comes from your prenatal supplement.

** You need 30 mg of iron daily, but some of that comes from your prenatal supplement.

— WEEK 11 —

Appointments:

Date _____ Time _____

Date _____ Time _____

Remember to find out if _____

_____

_____

Goals:

Next week I will _____

_____

❧

People may tell you not to eat liver, an excellent source of iron, because it is high in cholesterol and may contain harmful substances. If you like liver, eating it once or twice a month is fine. Anyone can eat a high cholesterol food once in a while without concern. And though the liver does help rid the body of harmful substances, it does not store them; instead it helps the body excrete those substances or store them in fat.

❧

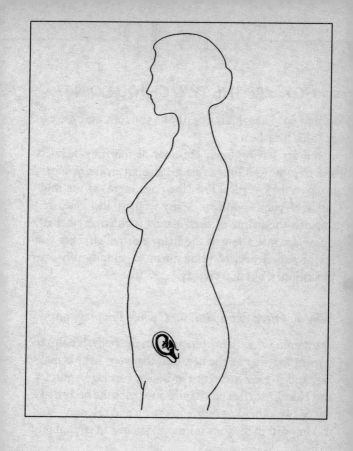

WEEK 12

HOW ARE THE TWO OF YOU DOING?

Your baby has all his tiny fingers and toes, and you can hear his heartbeat.

You are having fewer episodes of morning sickness and nausea. Your breasts are getting larger, and you may notice a dark vertical line (the linea nigra) at the midpoint of your abdomen. Many women also get a red tinge to the palms of their hands (palmar erythema). These are just a few of the many normal changes you might experience. Mention them to your health care practitioner, but don't worry.

Why do I need extra vitamin C while I'm pregnant?

Vitamin C has many functions in the body. It helps to cement together all the new cells that your baby is making, and it gives structure to bones, cartilage, muscles, and blood vessels. The vitamin also helps the body make use of two other key nutrients—iron and calcium—and it is important for your immune system and your ability to heal.

Everyone knows orange juice is an excellent source of vitamin C. Here are some other good sources:

baked potato	papaya
broccoli	persimmon
Brussels sprouts	red and green peppers
cantaloupe	spinach
cauliflower	strawberries
collard greens	tangerine
fresh pineapple	tomato and tomato juice
grapefruit	vitamin C–fortified juice
and grapefruit juice	watermelon
guava	

Aim for 2 servings of vitamin C–rich foods each day.

WEEK 12

PREGNANCY FOOD CHECKLIST

Goals:
- 2–3 servings of protein-rich foods
- 3 servings of calcium-rich foods
- 5 or more fruits and vegetables
- 6 or more servings of breads, grains, and cereals

	Calories	Protein	Vit C	Folic Acid	Calcium	Iron
Breakfast						
Subtotal	___	___	___	___	___	___
Snack						
Subtotal	___	___	___	___	___	___
Lunch						
Subtotal	___	___	___	___	___	___
Snack						
Subtotal	___	___	___	___	___	___
Dinner						
Subtotal	___	___	___	___	___	___
Snack						
Subtotal	___	___	___	___	___	___
Daily total	___	___	___	___	___	___
Daily Nutrient Goals	2200	60	70	300–400*	1000	10–15**

* You need 600 mcg of folic acid daily, but some of that comes from your prenatal supplement.

** You need 30 mg of iron daily, but some of that comes from your prenatal supplement.

WEEK 12

Appointments:

Date _____ Time _____

Date _____ Time _____

Remember to find out if _____

_____

_____

Goals:

Next week I will _____

_____

My weight is _____

If your pregnancy was an unexpected but wonderful surprise, you are not alone—more than half of all pregnancies in the United States are unplanned.

WEEK 13

HOW ARE THE TWO OF YOU DOING?

Your baby is the size of a peach. From here on, her tissues and organs will grow and develop rapidly. Her face now looks like that of a tiny human, and the genitalia are developed enough to tell little girls from boys.

You are in the "easy" part of pregnancy right now. Morning sickness and nausea have passed. Your tummy is beginning to bulge like a smooth ball, but it's not big enough to get in your way. You feel good. You're happy, and your old energy level is back. This isn't going to be so hard after all!

I love my morning cup of coffee. Do I have to give it up?

The coffee is not the problem, but the caffeine is troublesome. If you drink decaf (caffeine-free), there's no need to change. If you drink regular coffee, we'd suggest sticking with one morning cup. You can cut the caffeine by making your morning coffee with half decaf and half regular coffee; some brands sell a half-and-half mixture.

Caffeine is a chemical stimulant found in coffee, tea, soda, cocoa, chocolate, and some medications. Coffee, tea, and soda contain the most. Almost all the caffeine taken in is absorbed and can cross the placenta. Pregnant women eliminate caffeine much more slowly. The jury is still out on caffeine—it does not appear to cause serious problems in pregnancy, but more than 3 cups of coffee a day may cause a slightly lower birth weight.

We suggest 1 or 2 caffeine-containing drinks a day and spacing out your intake so that your body has a chance to clear the caffeine before you have more. Caffeine-containing drinks are usually just flavorful, pleasurable choices. If you cut back or even cut them out, you won't be losing any important key nutrients.

WEEK 13

PREGNANCY FOOD CHECKLIST

Goals:
- 2–3 servings of protein-rich foods
- 3 servings of calcium-rich foods
- 5 or more fruits and vegetables
- 6 or more servings of breads, grains, and cereals

	Calories	Protein	Vit C	Folic Acid	Calcium	Iron
Breakfast						
Subtotal	____	____	____	____	____	____
Snack						
Subtotal	____	____	____	____	____	____
Lunch						
Subtotal	____	____	____	____	____	____
Snack						
Subtotal	____	____	____	____	____	____
Dinner						
Subtotal	____	____	____	____	____	____
Snack						
Subtotal	____	____	____	____	____	____
Daily total	____	____	____	____	____	____
Daily Nutrient Goals	2200	60	70	300–400*	1000	10–15**

* You need 600 mcg of folic acid daily, but some of that comes from your prenatal supplement.
** You need 30 mg of iron daily, but some of that comes from your prenatal supplement.

WEEK 13

Appointments:

Date _____ Time _____

Date _____ Time _____

Remember to find out if _____

_____

_____

Goals:

Next week I will _____

_____

❊

Nearly 20% of all pregnant women are bothered by itching. They have no rash, hives, or bumps; they just itch. Ask your health care practitioner for the name of a cooling lotion that may help. Don't worry about your baby—he's not bothered by this at all.

❊

WEEK 14

HOW ARE THE TWO OF YOU DOING?

Your baby is about the size of your fist, and his neck is getting longer so that the head no longer appears to sit right on his shoulders.

You can easily tell you're pregnant by the appearance of your lower abdomen. Women who have been pregnant before often show earlier, carry lower, and feel bigger than first-time moms.

Why is it so important not to drink any alcohol while I'm pregnant?

Drinking large amounts of alcohol while you are pregnant can cause serious damage to your developing baby. Almost everyone knows this. What they don't know is how much is too much. Even 1 to 2 drinks a day will increase the risk for lower birth weight, which in turn increases your baby's risk for other health problems.

Alcohol freely crosses the placenta, so your baby is drinking along with you. Unfortunately, her immature liver cannot efficiently break down alcohol the way you can, so this potentially damaging substance circulates through her delicate developing body for a long time before it's removed.

Here's the best advice: to be perfectly safe, don't drink any alcohol at all during pregnancy.

WEEK 14

PREGNANCY FOOD CHECKLIST

Goals:
- 2–3 servings of protein-rich foods
- 3 servings of calcium-rich foods
- 5 or more fruits and vegetables
- 6 or more servings of breads, grains, and cereals

	Calories	Protein	Vit C	Folic Acid	Calcium	Iron
Breakfast						
Subtotal	____	____	____	____	____	____
Snack						
Subtotal	____	____	____	____	____	____
Lunch						
Subtotal	____	____	____	____	____	____
Snack						
Subtotal	____	____	____	____	____	____
Dinner						
Subtotal	____	____	____	____	____	____
Snack						
Subtotal	____	____	____	____	____	____
Daily total	____	____	____	____	____	____
Daily Nutrient Goals	2200	60	70	300–400*	1000	10–15**

* You need 600 mcg of folic acid daily, but some of that comes from your prenatal supplement.

** You need 30 mg of iron daily, but some of that comes from your prenatal supplement,

Appointments:

Date _____ Time _____

Date _____ Time _____

Remember to find out if _____

_____

_____

Goals:

Next week I will _____

_____

Don't put your baby at risk. A recent study showed that 15% of college-educated women drank alcohol while they were pregnant.

WEEK 15

HOW ARE THE TWO OF YOU DOING?

Your baby is about the size of a softball. If you could peek inside your uterus, you might see him sucking his thumb. His body is covered with fine hair (lanugo), and his skin is so thin that you can see his tiny blood vessels. His entire skeleton, though tiny, is formed.

You look pregnant now, and it's hard to find something in your closet that's comfortable. Many women borrow their partner's shirts and sweats at this point. It's time to go on a maternity shopping spree.

I have an incredible craving for popcorn. Is it okay to eat it every day?

Pregnancy, pickles, and ice cream seem to go hand in hand. Every pregnant woman has a story about a food she craved and another she couldn't bear to go near: 80% of all pregnant women crave certain foods, while 50% find some foods intolerable. Normal changes in taste and smell along with cultural beliefs explain some cravings. Experts agree that cravings do occur during pregnancy, but they aren't quite sure why.

It's okay to indulge your craving for popcorn—

unbuttered is best—but don't go overboard and ignore other important foods. Stay away from any foods that bother you. If you crave nonfood items, which might contain harmful substances, talk this over with your health care practitioner.

WEEK 15

PREGNANCY FOOD CHECKLIST

Goals:
- 2–3 servings of protein-rich foods
- 3 servings of calcium-rich foods
- 5 or more fruits and vegetables
- 6 or more servings of breads, grains, and cereals

	Calories	Protein	Vit C	Folic Acid	Calcium	Iron
Breakfast						
Subtotal	_____	_____	_____	_____	_____	_____
Snack						
Subtotal	_____	_____	_____	_____	_____	_____
Lunch						
Subtotal	_____	_____	_____	_____	_____	_____
Snack						
Subtotal	_____	_____	_____	_____	_____	_____
Dinner						
Subtotal	_____	_____	_____	_____	_____	_____
Snack						
Subtotal	_____	_____	_____	_____	_____	_____
Daily total	_____	_____	_____	_____	_____	_____
Daily Nutrient Goals	2200	60	70	300–400*	1000	10–15**

* You need 600 mcg of folic acid daily, but some of that comes from your prenatal supplement.

** You need 30 mg of iron daily, but some of that comes from your prenatal supplement.

WEEK 15

Appointments:

Date _____ Time _____

Date _____ Time _____

Remember to find out if _____

_____

_____

Goals:

Next week I will _____

_____

❋

You may have an occasional nosebleed or headache. This is simply a sign that your body is adjusting to the increased blood volume and vessel tension. Neither is a problem to worry about, but tell your health care practitioner if either occurs.

❋

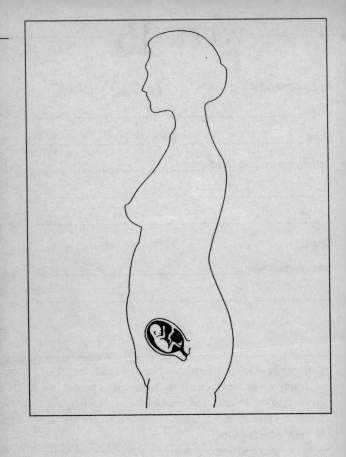

WEEK 16

HOW ARE THE TWO OF YOU DOING?

Your baby is actively moving around.

You might have felt this movement. If you haven't, don't worry, you will soon. Many women compare this early movement to fluttering or blowing bubbles. Your little one is making himself known!

I've read that I should eat balanced meals while I'm pregnant. What exactly is a balanced meal?

Balanced meals include foods from most of the food groups—bread or cereals, fruits and vegetables, milk or other dairy foods, and meat or other protein-rich foods. Another way to achieve balance is to eat a "colorful plate." When you select a variety of different-colored foods, you increase your intake of important vitamins and minerals. Each day aim for the serving recommendations listed above the Pregnancy Food Checklist, and stretch the boundaries of your food experiences by trying new choices and new tastes. Don't always reach for an apple or drink only orange juice. Try instead papayas, raisins, pineapple or mango juice. You have the best reason in the world for making healthy food choices.

WEEK 16

PREGNANCY FOOD CHECKLIST

Goals:
- 2–3 servings of protein-rich foods
- 3 servings of calcium-rich foods
- 5 or more fruits and vegetables
- 6 or more servings of breads, grains, and cereals

	Calories	Protein	Vit C	Folic Acid	Calcium	Iron
Breakfast						
Subtotal	___	___	___	___	___	___
Snack						
Subtotal	___	___	___	___	___	___
Lunch						
Subtotal	___	___	___	___	___	___
Snack						
Subtotal	___	___	___	___	___	___
Dinner						
Subtotal	___	___	___	___	___	___
Snack						
Subtotal	___	___	___	___	___	___
Daily total	___	___	___	___	___	___
Daily Nutrient Goals	2200	60	70	300–400*	1000	10–15**

* You need 600 mcg of folic acid daily, but some of that comes from your prenatal supplement.

** You need 30 mg of iron daily, but some of that comes from your prenatal supplement.

Appointments:

Date _____ Time _____

Date _____ Time _____

Remember to find out if _____

_____

_____

Goals:

Next week I will _____

_____

My weight is _____

Because all foods contain a mixture of nutrients, those that are excellent sources of a key nutrient will provide many other nutrients as well. Milk, an excellent source of the key nutrient calcium, is also rich in protein, vitamin D, vitamin A, and potassium.

HOW ARE THE TWO OF YOU DOING?

Your baby is the size of your hand when it is open wide, and she is starting to develop body fat.

You have gained 5 to 10 pounds by now, and when your partner gives you a hug, he can feel your baby in the middle.

Is it safe to use the microwave while I'm pregnant?

Microwave ovens are among the safest appliances in the home. The radiation used for heating is the same as radio-frequency radiation, not X-rays. Because foods heat faster at lower temperatures than in a broiler or oven, fewer nutrients are destroyed when food is cooked in a microwave oven.

Accidents can occur, however, when food is over-heated in the microwave, because it can splatter or spit. Always cut slits in the food wrap to let steam escape, use a pot holder to remove food from the oven, and re-move the lid in the direction away from you. Plastic particles from food containers and wraps can melt into food and may interfere with hormone function. It's easy to avoid this problem by heating in microwave-safe containers.

Safe to use	*Best to avoid*
glass, like Pyrex	leftover margarine tubs
ceramic glass,	take-out food containers
like Corning Ware	plastic meat trays
microwave-safe rigid plastic	plastic containers
plastic wraps, like Glad Wrap	not labeled
wax paper	"microwave safe"
unprinted paper towels	cling-type plastic wrap,
plastic food storage bags	like Reynolds
	and Saran Wrap
	grocery store plastic bags

WEEK 17

PREGNANCY FOOD CHECKLIST

Goals:
- 2–3 servings of protein-rich foods
- 3 servings of calcium-rich foods
- 5 or more fruits and vegetables
- 6 or more servings of breads, grains, and cereals

	Calories	Protein	Vit C	Folic Acid	Calcium	Iron
Breakfast						
Subtotal	____	____	____	____	____	____
Snack						
Subtotal	____	____	____	____	____	____
Lunch						
Subtotal	____	____	____	____	____	____
Snack						
Subtotal	____	____	____	____	____	____
Dinner						
Subtotal	____	____	____	____	____	____
Snack						
Subtotal	____	____	____	____	____	____
Daily total	____	____	____	____	____	____
Daily Nutrient Goals	2200	60	70	300–400*	1000	10–15**

* You need 600 mcg of folic acid daily, but some of that comes from your prenatal supplement.
** You need 30 mg of iron daily, but some of that comes from your prenatal supplement.

WEEK 17

Appointments:

Date _____ Time _____

Date _____ Time _____

Remember to find out if _____

_____

_____

Goals:

Next week I will _____

_____

❀

Your baby depends on you to maintain his correct body temperature. Many experts feel it is unwise for pregnant women to use hot tubs and saunas. Try instead a swim or a long, leisurely shower.

❀

WEEK 18

HOW ARE THE TWO OF YOU DOING?

Your baby weighs about 5 ounces and is actively doing somersaults in your uterus.

You may get an occasional backache as your uterus grows out in front of you and changes your center of gravity. Get off your feet often during the day, and whenever possible lie on your side to relieve the pressure on your back.

Is it okay to exercise while I'm pregnant?

There was a time when pregnant women were forbidden to exercise. Today there are classes especially designed for working out during pregnancy. If you have been active all along, keep it up. Swimming, bicycling, and even jogging are all encouraged. Keeping in shape physically will aid your digestion, improve your sleep, and help you during labor. If you were not active before pregnancy, go easy. Talk to your health care practitioner and start with something simple like a daily walk.

WEEK 18

PREGNANCY FOOD CHECKLIST

Goals:
- 2–3 servings of protein-rich foods
- 3 servings of calcium-rich foods
- 5 or more fruits and vegetables
- 6 or more servings of breads, grains, and cereals

		Calories	Protein	Vit C	Folic Acid	Calcium	Iron
Breakfast							
	Subtotal	____	____	____	____	____	____
Snack							
	Subtotal	____	____	____	____	____	____
Lunch							
	Subtotal	____	____	____	____	____	____
Snack							
	Subtotal	____	____	____	____	____	____
Dinner							
	Subtotal	____	____	____	____	____	____
Snack							
	Subtotal	____	____	____	____	____	____
	Daily total	____	____	____	____	____	____
Daily Nutrient Goals		2200	60	70	300–400*	1000	10–15**

* You need 600 mcg of folic acid daily, but some of that comes from your prenatal supplement.
** You need 30 mg of iron daily, but some of that comes from your prenatal supplement.

WEEK 18

Appointments:

Date _____ Time _____

Date _____ Time _____

Remember to find out if _____

_____

_____

Goals:

Next week I will _____

_____

❀

All your baby's nutrients and oxygen are delivered from
your bloodstream across the placenta to your baby.
Though the circulation of your blood and your baby's
comes very close, there is no direct connection.

❀

WEEK 19

HOW ARE THE TWO OF YOU DOING?

Your baby has gained almost 2 ounces since last week. She now weighs about 7 ounces.

You have gained between 8 and 14 pounds by now. Why, you wonder, when your baby weighs only 7 ounces? Remember that many other things are changing to accommodate your pregnancy. Your breasts have gotten bigger, your uterus is enlarging, your blood volume has increased, the placenta has developed, and you now have about 11 ounces of amniotic fluid in your uterus.

Sometimes I feel very dizzy. Is there anything I can do to avoid this?

Feeling dizzy is common during pregnancy. It can be caused by your enlarging uterus putting pressure on your heart vessels when you lie down, especially if you recline on your back. Sometimes it happens when you get up quickly. Lying on your side and getting up slowly may solve the problem.

Dizziness can also be caused by low blood sugar (hypoglycemia). You can often solve this problem, or at least minimize it, by not going for long periods without eat-

nd by not skipping meals. When you are on the
[go] carry a piece of fruit, some raisins, a cereal bar, or
graham crackers for a quick blood sugar boost.

Let your health care practitioner know if these simple
solutions aren't working.

WEEK 19

PREGNANCY FOOD CHECKLIST

Goals:
- 2–3 servings of protein-rich foods
- 3 servings of calcium-rich foods
- 5 or more fruits and vegetables
- 6 or more servings of breads, grains, and cereals

	Calories	Protein	Vit C	Folic Acid	Calcium	Iron
Breakfast						
Subtotal	____	____	____	____	____	____
Snack						
Subtotal	____	____	____	____	____	____
Lunch						
Subtotal	____	____	____	____	____	____
Snack						
Subtotal	____	____	____	____	____	____
Dinner						
Subtotal	____	____	____	____	____	____
Snack						
Subtotal	____	____	____	____	____	____
Daily total	____	____	____	____	____	____
Daily Nutrient Goals	2200	60	70	300–400*	1000	10–15**

* You need 600 mcg of folic acid daily, but some of that comes from your prenatal supplement.

** You need 30 mg of iron daily, but some of that comes from your prenatal supplement.

— WEEK 19 —

Appointments:

Date _____ Time _____

Date _____ Time _____

Remember to find out if _____

_____

_____

Goals:

Next week I will _____

_____

It's important to share with your partner the miracle that's happening in your body. Let him feel the baby move, and take him to meet your health care practitioner so he can hear his baby's heartbeat.

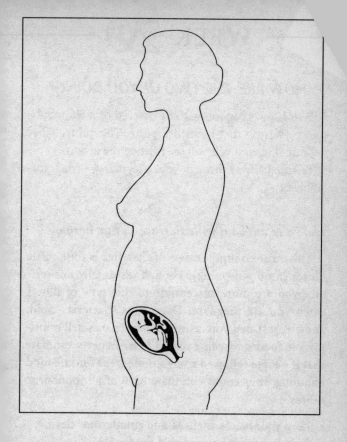

— WEEK 20 —

HOW ARE THE TWO OF YOU DOING?

Your baby is beginning to be covered by a white substance (vernix) that looks like paste. This protects her delicate skin, and you will see it when she is born.

You are halfway through your pregnancy—congratulations!

I had a recent bout with diarrhea. Is that normal?

The most common cause of diarrhea is foodborne illness (food poisoning). Though it's usually not serious, you are more susceptible to this type of illness when you are pregnant. Organisms (bacteria, mold, and viruses) that you cannot see, taste, or smell multiply on food and can cause illness. Experts estimate that if people followed a few simple steps for safe food handling, they could eliminate 85% of all foodborne illness.

- Keep your hands, utensils, and countertops clean.
- Keep hot foods hot and cold foods cold.
- Keep raw foods and cooked foods separate during preparation.

- Cook all food thoroughly; don't eat undercooked or rare foods.
- When in doubt throw it out.

WEEK 20

PREGNANCY FOOD CHECKLIST

Goals:
- 2–3 servings of protein-rich foods
- 3 servings of calcium-rich foods
- 5 or more fruits and vegetables
- 6 or more servings of breads, grains, and cereals

	Calories	Protein	Vit C	Folic Acid	Calcium	Iron
Breakfast						
Subtotal	___	___	___	___	___	___
Snack						
Subtotal	___	___	___	___	___	___
Lunch						
Subtotal	___	___	___	___	___	___
Snack						
Subtotal	___	___	___	___	___	___
Dinner						
Subtotal	___	___	___	___	___	___
Snack						
Subtotal	___	___	___	___	___	___
Daily total	___	___	___	___	___	___
Daily Nutrient Goals	2200	60	70	300–400*	1000	10–15**

* You need 600 mcg of folic acid daily, but some of that comes from your prenatal supplement.

** You need 30 mg of iron daily, but some of that comes from your prenatal supplement.

Appointments:

Date _____ Time _____

Date _____ Time _____

Remember to find out if _____

_____

_____

Goals:

Next week I will _____

_____

My weight is _____

❀

It's normal to have an increased vaginal discharge or se-
cretion (leukorrhea) that may be thick white or yellowish.
It is not an infection and nothing to worry about.

❀

WEEK 21

HOW ARE THE TWO OF YOU DOING?

Your baby weighs about 11 ounces and is the size of a large banana.

You have lost your waistline and you definitely look pregnant.

I like sweet foods, but my friend told me to stop eating white sugar while I'm pregnant. Is that necessary?

Sugar is sugar whether it's white, brown, powdered, honey, molasses, or maple sugar. None is better or worse than another. It's estimated that we eat 32 teaspoons of sugar a day. Some sweets—like fruits, cereal, fruit drinks, and hot cocoa—are good for you. Others—like candy, cake, and soda—may crowd out more nourishing foods by providing a lot of calories but very few nutrients. Choose wisely, and make sweets count.

Instead of this sweet	Try a healthier sweet
candy bar	granola or cereal bar
pastry	raisin bread
ice cream	fruit sorbet

hot fudge sundae	banana split with fruit and nut topping
soda	fruit juice or nectar
cookies	graham crackers or fruit bars
cake	banana bread or carrot cake
gummy candy	peanut butter cups

— WEEK 21 —

PREGNANCY FOOD CHECKLIST

Goals:
- 2–3 servings of protein-rich foods
- 3 servings of calcium-rich foods
- 5 or more fruits and vegetables
- 6 or more servings of breads, grains, and cereals

	Calories	Protein	Vit C	Folic Acid	Calcium	Iron
Breakfast						
Subtotal	____	____	____	____	____	____
Snack						
Subtotal	____	____	____	____	____	____
Lunch						
Subtotal	____	____	____	____	____	____
Snack						
Subtotal	____	____	____	____	____	____
Dinner						
Subtotal	____	____	____	____	____	____
Snack						
Subtotal	____	____	____	____	____	____
Daily total	____	____	____	____	____	____
Daily Nutrient Goals	2200	60	70	300–400*	1000	10–15**

* You need 600 mcg of folic acid daily, but some of that comes from your prenatal supplement.
** You need 30 mg of iron daily, but some of that comes from your prenatal supplement.

WEEK 21

Appointments:

Date _____ Time _____

Date _____ Time _____

Remember to find out if _____

_____

_____

Goals:

Next week I will _____

_____

❀

Sweetened ready-to-eat cereal is a healthy, tasty, and quick
treat. All varieties are made from a grain (some are whole
grain), low in fat, and fortified with iron and folic acid, 2
key nutrients.

❀

WEEK 22

HOW ARE THE TWO OF YOU DOING?

Your baby's digestive system has developed, and he is swallowing amniotic fluid. Researchers believe this may be one way your baby gets some of the key nutrients needed for growth and development, and it may prepare the digestive system to function after birth.

You are having fun being pregnant. Your abdomen isn't large enough to get in the way, you can still bend and sit comfortably, you feel good, and you are happy.

I've been told to stop drinking diet soda while I'm pregnant because it can cause cancer. Is that true?

Diet sodas that contain saccharin, one type of sugar substitute, must carry a warning label because some research has shown that huge amounts might promote bladder cancer in male rats. Many experts feel these findings are not related to the cause of human bladder cancer. Once again the jury is out, but we suggest very limited use of saccharin (Sweet'n Low, Sugar Twin) during pregnancy because this sweetener crosses the placenta and your baby clears it very slowly.

There are 3 other approved sugar substitutes:

Acesulfame-K (Sunett) is considered safe to use during pregnancy. It's made from a naturally occurring acid combined with a mineral, and it's found in diet sodas like Pepsi One.

Aspartame (NutraSweet, Equal, NatraTaste) is made by combining two protein fragments that occur naturally in many foods we eat. It is safe to use during pregnancy. All foods that contain it must carry a warning label because a very small part of the population with a rare genetic condition cannot digest one of the protein fragments used to make this sweetener.

Sucralose (Splenda) is the only sugar substitute made from sugar so it is safe to use during pregnancy. It is used to sweeten drinks like Diet RC cola and Diet Veryfine juice.

Like sugar, sugar substitutes offer no key nutrients so you lose nothing by limiting or eliminating them while you are pregnant. On the other hand, using small amounts carries no risk.

PREGNANCY FOOD CHECKLIST

Goals:
- 2–3 servings of protein-rich foods
- 3 servings of calcium-rich foods
- 5 or more fruits and vegetables
- 6 or more servings of breads, grains, and cereals

	Calories	Protein	Vit C	Folic Acid	Calcium	Iron
Breakfast						
Subtotal	____	____	____	____	____	____
Snack						
Subtotal	____	____	____	____	____	____
Lunch						
Subtotal	____	____	____	____	____	____
Snack						
Subtotal	____	____	____	____	____	____
Dinner						
Subtotal	____	____	____	____	____	____
Snack						
Subtotal	____	____	____	____	____	____
Daily total	____	____	____	____	____	____
Daily Nutrient Goals	2200	60	70	300–400*	1000	10–15**

* You need 600 mcg of folic acid daily, but some of that comes from your prenatal supplement.
** You need 30 mg of iron daily, but some of that comes from your prenatal supplement.

WEEK 22

Appointments:

Date _____ Time _____

Date _____ Time _____

Remember to find out if _____

_____

_____

Goals:

Next week I will _____

_____

Your health care practitioner may begin measuring your belly with a tape measure. This is a way to monitor the size and growth of your baby. You grow about 1 centimeter each week; your measurement will closely equal your week of pregnancy.

WEEK 23

HOW ARE THE TWO OF YOU DOING?

Your baby is about the size of a small doll, and she is getting plumper every week.

You are back in the bathroom every half hour because your expanding uterus is putting a lot of pressure on your bladder.

My partner bugs me to eat breakfast. Do I have to? I'm always so late in the morning.

The word breakfast means "to break the fast." Neither you nor your baby has eaten since last night. It's wise to eat something in the morning, but we can appreciate how hectic mornings can be. A recent survey showed that people are looking for low-maintenance breakfasts that they can eat in the car, on the train, at their desk, or even while getting dressed.

What do you like to eat—bagels, cereal bars, yogurt, fruit, toaster pastry, instant breakfast drink, crackers and cheese? All of these foods are portable. Don't be afraid to be adventurous—try pizza, dinner leftovers, a sandwich, a milk shake. Breakfast can be anything you like, so long as it provides some of the key nutrients and gets you and your baby off to a good start.

WEEK 23

PREGNANCY FOOD CHECKLIST

Goals:
- 2–3 servings of protein-rich foods
- 3 servings of calcium-rich foods
- 5 or more fruits and vegetables
- 6 or more servings of breads, grains, and cereals

	Calories	Protein	Vit C	Folic Acid	Calcium	Iron
Breakfast						
Subtotal	___	___	___	___	___	___
Snack						
Subtotal	___	___	___	___	___	___
Lunch						
Subtotal	___	___	___	___	___	___
Snack						
Subtotal	___	___	___	___	___	___
Dinner						
Subtotal	___	___	___	___	___	___
Snack						
Subtotal	___	___	___	___	___	___
Daily total	___	___	___	___	___	___
Daily Nutrient Goals	2200	60	70	300–400*	1000	10–15**

* You need 600 mcg of folic acid daily, but some of that comes from your prenatal supplement.

** You need 30 mg of iron daily, but some of that comes from your prenatal supplement.

WEEK 23

Appointments:

Date _____ Time _____

Date _____ Time _____

Remember to find out if _____

_____

_____

Goals:

Next week I will _____

_____

❋

At times you may feel like a little old lady, unable to stand up quickly and creaking when you bend or walk. This happens because the hormone relaxin is "relaxing" the ligaments around your pelvis and hips so that they will stretch more easily during labor.

❋

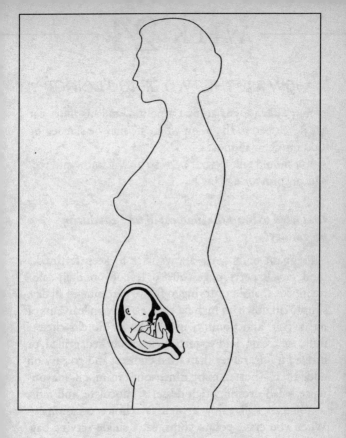

WEEK 24

HOW ARE THE TWO OF YOU DOING?

Your baby weighs at least a pound, and his inner ear has developed to the point where he may be startled by loud music or sounds.

You should talk to your baby so he will know and recognize your voice at birth.

Do I need to limit the amount of fat I eat during pregnancy?

Pregnant or not, it's always wise to keep fat intake moderate. Experts suggest 30% or less of your daily calorie intake. Instead of trying to figure percentages all day, simply cut down on high fat choices. Rely on lean cuts of meat, fish, and poultry; use lowfat or nonfat cheese, milk, ice cream, and yogurt; stick with baked, grilled, or broiled foods, rather than fried choices; and go easy on added fats—butter, margarine, sour cream, oil, mayonnaise, salad dressing, rich desserts, chocolate, and nuts.

You can still enjoy a high fat choice occasionally. When you crave potato chips, eat a single-serving bag. Dying for french fries? Eat a small order. Can't resist chocolate cake for dessert? Split a serving with your partner. Want a candy bar? Have a snack-size bar.

WEEK 24

PREGNANCY FOOD CHECKLIST

Goals:
- 2–3 servings of protein-rich foods
- 3 servings of calcium-rich foods
- 5 or more fruits and vegetables
- 6 or more servings of breads, grains, and cereals

	Calories	Protein	Vit C	Folic Acid	Calcium	Iron
Breakfast						
Subtotal	___	___	___	___	___	___
Snack						
Subtotal	___	___	___	___	___	___
Lunch						
Subtotal	___	___	___	___	___	___
Snack						
Subtotal	___	___	___	___	___	___
Dinner						
Subtotal	___	___	___	___	___	___
Snack						
Subtotal	___	___	___	___	___	___
Daily total	___	___	___	___	___	___
Daily Nutrient Goals	2200	60	70	300–400*	1000	10–15**

* You need 600 mcg of folic acid daily, but some of that comes from your prenatal supplement.

** You need 30 mg of iron daily, but some of that comes from your prenatal supplement.

— WEEK 24 —

Appointments:

Date _____ Time _____

Date _____ Time _____

Remember to find out if _____

_____

_____

Goals:

Next week I will _____

_____

My weight is _____

❁

Foods high in fat are often high in cholesterol, too. When you eat moderate amounts of fat, you automatically eat moderate amounts of cholesterol.

❁

WEEK 25

HOW ARE THE TWO OF YOU DOING?

Your baby can swallow, taste, hear, and regulate her body temperature, but she still depends on your support to continue to grow.

You have entered your last trimester—the home stretch! You feel a little uncomfortable, and you're tired of waiting, but you are also reassured by your baby's frequent movements. Each passing day brings you closer to your due date.

Should I get my cholesterol tested while I'm pregnant?

When you are pregnant your cholesterol level goes up as a natural response to pregnancy. If you have your cholesterol values screened now, without knowing this, you might be alarmed by these higher than normal levels. Values will return to pre-pregnancy levels within a few months after your baby is born.

Most people think of cholesterol as a harmful substance that can lead to heart disease. You might be surprised to find out that there is cholesterol in every cell in your body and your baby's body. It is essential for proper development. You get your needed cholesterol in food, and you make it in the liver. When you make healthy food choices and eat moderate amounts of high fat foods, you are automatically eating a moderate amount of cholesterol.

WEEK 25

PREGNANCY FOOD CHECKLIST

Goals:
- 2–3 servings of protein-rich foods
- 3 servings of calcium-rich foods
- 5 or more fruits and vegetables
- 6 or more servings of breads, grains, and cereals

	Calories	Protein	Vit C	Folic Acid	Calcium	Iron
Breakfast						
Subtotal	___	___	___	___	___	___
Snack						
Subtotal	___	___	___	___	___	___
Lunch						
Subtotal	___	___	___	___	___	___
Snack						
Subtotal	___	___	___	___	___	___
Dinner						
Subtotal	___	___	___	___	___	___
Snack						
Subtotal	___	___	___	___	___	___
Daily total	___	___	___	___	___	___
Daily Nutrient Goals	2200	60	70	300–400*	1000	10–15**

* You need 600 mcg of folic acid daily, but some of that comes from your prenatal supplement.

** You need 30 mg of iron daily, but some of that comes from your prenatal supplement.

WEEK 25

Appointments:

Date _____ Time _____

Date _____ Time _____

Remember to find out if _____

_____

_____

Goals:

Next week I will _____

_____

❀

Over the next 12 weeks your baby will grow very rapidly. You could easily gain a pound a week. Don't worry, this weight is a combination of your growing baby and the systems needed to support him. Women who eat well throughout pregnancy and gain the appropriate amount of weight are more likely to have healthy babies. Take good care of both of you.

❀

WEEK 26

HOW ARE THE TWO OF YOU DOING?

Your baby weighs almost 2 pounds, and although he is still very active, he has quiet periods too. Unfortunately they rarely occur at night.

You are having difficulty sleeping, and you may feel breathless as your growing baby pushes your abdomen up against your diaphragm.

I'm constipated. Should I take a laxative?

Talk to your health care practitioner before you take a laxative. She might recommend prune juice, which contains a natural laxative. Sometimes just adding more fiber to your meals will solve the problem.

Fiber is the part of plants we cannot digest. Why, then, do we need it?

Your digestive tract is one of the largest muscles in your body, and like any muscle, it needs exercise, especially toward the end of pregnancy when it is sandwiched between your backbone and your growing baby. Moving fiber along the intestines exercises the muscle. Fiber also absorbs water, making your stools softer and easier to pass.

For a fiber boost

Instead of this:	*Try this:*
white bread	rye bread
white rice	brown rice
pasta	whole wheat pasta
jellied cranberry sauce	whole cranberry sauce
apple juice	whole apple
tomato juice	whole tomato
mashed potatoes	baked potato with skin
farina	oatmeal
corn flakes	bran flakes
sugar cookies	fig newtons
jelly	whole berry jelly
chocolate candy	chocolate-covered raisins
cheese pizza	vegetable pizza
pretzels	whole wheat pretzels

— WEEK 26 —

PREGNANCY FOOD CHECKLIST

Goals:
- 2–3 servings of protein-rich foods
- 3 servings of calcium-rich foods
- 5 or more fruits and vegetables
- 6 or more servings of breads, grains, and cereals

	Calories	Protein	Vit C	Folic Acid	Calcium	Iron
Breakfast						
Subtotal	____	____	____	____	____	____
Snack						
Subtotal	____	____	____	____	____	____
Lunch						
Subtotal	____	____	____	____	____	____
Snack						
Subtotal	____	____	____	____	____	____
Dinner						
Subtotal	____	____	____	____	____	____
Snack						
Subtotal	____	____	____	____	____	____
Daily total	____	____	____	____	____	____
Daily Nutrient Goals	2200	60	70	300–400*	1000	10–15**

* You need 600 mcg of folic acid daily, but some of that comes from your prenatal supplement.

** You need 30 mg of iron daily, but some of that comes from your prenatal supplement.

WEEK 26

Appointments:

Date _____ Time _____

Date _____ Time _____

Remember to find out if _____

_____

_____

Goals:

Next week I will _____

_____

❁

A large glass of juice, seltzer, or water with a bowl of popcorn makes a tasty and nutritious after-dinner snack. It's also a great way to add fiber and relieve constipation. It's important to drink plenty of fluids when you eat extra fiber.

❁

WEEK 27

HOW ARE THE TWO OF YOU DOING?

Your baby has begun to open and close his eyes.

You are dying of the heat while everyone around you is freezing. In the last trimester your basal metabolic rate (the rate at which calories are burned for energy when your body is at rest) increases. This helps you meet your baby's increased demands for growth and gives you a spurt of energy to get through the final sprint before delivery. Unfortunately, it also makes you less tolerant of heat—great for winter pregnancies, horrible in the summer.

I get full very quickly. I'm afraid I'm not eating enough.

At the end of pregnancy, the weight of your baby on your abdomen may make you feel full before you've finished your meal. Smaller meals and between-meal snacks may be a more comfortable and nourishing way to go.

- Consider each snack an extension of the last meal or a warm-up for the next one. Have toast and cocoa at mid-morning and a cup of soup late in the afternoon.
- Make snacks count. Fruits are rich in vitamins, whole

wheat breadsticks contain fiber, and yogurt is rich in calcium.

- If beverages fill you up too quickly, have your normal mealtime drink between meals.
- Be creative. Freeze fruit juice into ice pops for a refreshing summer snack or microwave a sweet potato for a nutrient-rich midwinter warm-up.

WEEK 27

PREGNANCY FOOD CHECKLIST

Goals:
- 2–3 servings of protein-rich foods
- 3 servings of calcium-rich foods
- 5 or more fruits and vegetables
- 6 or more servings of breads, grains, and cereals

	Calories	Protein	Vit C	Folic Acid	Calcium	Iron
Breakfast						
Subtotal	___	___	___	___	___	___
Snack						
Subtotal	___	___	___	___	___	___
Lunch						
Subtotal	___	___	___	___	___	___
Snack						
Subtotal	___	___	___	___	___	___
Dinner						
Subtotal	___	___	___	___	___	___
Snack						
Subtotal	___	___	___	___	___	___
Daily total	___	___	___	___	___	___
Daily Nutrient Goals	2200	60	70	300–400*	1000	10–15**

* You need 600 mcg of folic acid daily, but some of that comes from your prenatal supplement.

** You need 30 mg of iron daily, but some of that comes from your prenatal supplement.

Appointments:

Date _____ Time _____

Date _____ Time _____

Remember to find out if _____

_____

_____

Goals:

Next week I will _____

_____

❊

If you crave something sweet, stick with the best sweet choices: dried fruit, pudding, custard, bran muffin, baked apple, sweetened cereal.

❊

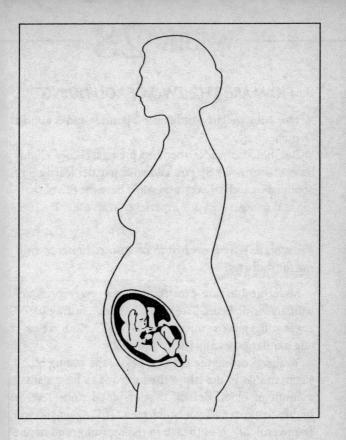

WEEK 28

HOW ARE THE TWO OF YOU DOING?

Your baby weighs a little over 2 pounds and is almost 16 inches long.

You should consider attending prenatal classes. Childbirth classes will help you and your partner learn more about labor and delivery, and you'll have the fun of sharing and comparing your experience with other couples.

I'm scared. Why is my health care practitioner testing me for diabetes?

Many health care practitioners test every pregnant woman for diabetes. The tests used are a fasting blood sugar and a glucose tolerance test (GTT). Both are easy, and neither poses any risk to your baby.

You stop eating the evening before the fasting blood sugar and go to the lab in the morning to have a small amount of blood drawn. If your blood sugar level is higher than normal, you will have a GTT. Again you will fast overnight, go to the lab in the morning, and have a small amount of blood drawn as a baseline. The technician will ask you to drink a beverage with a measured amount of sugar in it. Blood samples will be drawn at certain times over the next few hours to see how your body handles sugar.

Only 2% of all pregnant women develop a mild form of gestational, or pregnancy, diabetes. The chance of this happening to you is small, but the incidence increases as women get older. In almost all cases the problem can be handled by adjusting your diet, and it usually disappears after your baby is born.

WEEK 28

PREGNANCY FOOD CHECKLIST

Goals:
- 2–3 servings of protein-rich foods
- 3 servings of calcium-rich foods
- 5 or more fruits and vegetables
- 6 or more servings of breads, grains, and cereals

	Calories	Protein	Vit C	Folic Acid	Calcium	Iron
Breakfast						
Subtotal	___	___	___	___	___	___
Snack						
Subtotal	___	___	___	___	___	___
Lunch						
Subtotal	___	___	___	___	___	___
Snack						
Subtotal	___	___	___	___	___	___
Dinner						
Subtotal	___	___	___	___	___	___
Snack						
Subtotal	___	___	___	___	___	___
Daily total	___	___	___	___	___	___
Daily Nutrient Goals	2200	60	70	300–400*	1000	10–15**

* You need 600 mcg of folic acid daily, but some of that comes from your prenatal supplement.

** You need 30 mg of iron daily, but some of that comes from your prenatal supplement.

WEEK 28

Appointments:

Date _____ Time _____

Date _____ Time _____

Remember to find out if _____

_____

_____

Goals:

Next week I will _____

_____

My weight is _____

❁

Some pregnant women say they can feel their heart fluttering. A normal heart can easily deal with the extra work
of pregnancy, but your heartbeat may be more obvious as
your enlarging uterus pushes it up and slightly to the left.

❁

WEEK 29

HOW ARE THE TWO OF YOU DOING?

Your baby weighs over 2½ pounds and is growing quickly from week to week.

You have gained between 19 and 25 pounds.

WHO WILL DELIVER YOUR BABY?

Family practitioner—a doctor who cares for all your family needs and delivers babies too.

Obstetrician—a doctor who specializes in the care of pregnant women.

Perinatologist—a doctor who specializes in high-risk pregnancies (only 1 woman in 10 needs this care).

Nurse-midwife—a registered nurse with additional training and certification who cares for pregnant women and delivers babies.

Is there anything I can do for indigestion?

Gas and indigestion occur partly because your digestive tract is sandwiched in between your growing baby and your backbone, and partly because the hormone progesterone is relaxing the muscles in your uterus so it can stretch to fit your baby. This hormone relaxes your digestive system too, slowing it down and causing indigestion, burping, and sometimes embarrassing gas.

To reduce indigestion, try eating smaller, more frequent meals. Steer clear of fried and fatty foods, and don't eat right before bedtime. To reduce gas, eat slowly, chewing with your mouth closed, and sip beverages through a straw. Also, don't chew gum, which causes more swallowed air and makes the situation worse. Foods that contain a lot of air, like whipped cream and soda, can also increase gas and burping. Foods that cause gas vary from one person to another, but the most often reported are beans, onions, celery, cabbage, cauliflower, cucumbers, bananas, prune juice, bagels, and applesauce. If any of these bother you just cut them out for the next couple of weeks.

WEEK 29

PREGNANCY FOOD CHECKLIST

Goals:
- 2–3 servings of protein-rich foods
- 3 servings of calcium-rich foods
- 5 or more fruits and vegetables
- 6 or more servings of breads, grains, and cereals

	Calories	Protein	Vit C	Folic Acid	Calcium	Iron
Breakfast						
Subtotal	____	____	____	____	____	____
Snack						
Subtotal	____	____	____	____	____	____
Lunch						
Subtotal	____	____	____	____	____	____
Snack						
Subtotal	____	____	____	____	____	____
Dinner						
Subtotal	____	____	____	____	____	____
Snack						
Subtotal	____	____	____	____	____	____
Daily total	____	____	____	____	____	____
Daily Nutrient Goals	2200	60	70	300–400*	1000	10–15**

* You need 600 mcg of folic acid daily, but some of that comes from your prenatal supplement.
** You need 30 mg of iron daily, but some of that comes from your prenatal supplement.

WEEK 29

Appointments:

Date _____ Time _____

Date _____ Time _____

Remember to find out if _____

_____

_____

Goals:

Next week I will _____

_____

During the last 12 weeks of pregnancy your baby's bones are growing rapidly and hardening before birth. It's estimated that 250 to 300 milligrams of calcium a day are shuttled from your bloodstream through the placenta to your baby. Thirsty? Have a glass of milk.

HOW ARE THE TWO OF YOU DOING?

Your baby weighs almost 3 pounds and is 17 inches long.

You can't believe you still have 10 weeks to go, you feel like you're running out of room and couldn't possibly get any bigger. Your little one who is not so little anymore is pushing everything that used to be in place out of place. You feel pressure—in your rib cage, on your back and down your legs.

I'm not a vegetable eater. Can I get the same nutrients from fruits?

You aren't alone, between 1970 and 1996, Americans increased their vegetable intake by only half a serving (that's equal to a 1/4 cup!). You probably eat more vegetables than you realize—remember potatoes are a vegetable as is salad. Fruits and vegetables are both rich in vitamins and minerals. Some are great sources of one key nutrient but all contain at least a little of many necessary vitamins and minerals. Right now you are most concerned with the key nutrients.

These fruits are good sources of key nutrients:

Vitamin C	Folic Acid *	Iron *
orange juice	oranges	blueberries
grapefruit juice	orange juice	prune juice
papaya	cantaloupe	prunes
fresh pineapple	strawberries	raisins
cantaloupe		dried apricots
strawberries		
watermelon		

* These key nutrients are also found in your prenatal vitamin supplement.

WEEK 30

PREGNANCY FOOD CHECKLIST

Goals:
- 2–3 servings of protein-rich foods
- 3 servings of calcium-rich foods
- 5 or more fruits and vegetables
- 6 or more servings of breads, grains, and cereals

	Calories	Protein	Vit C	Folic Acid	Calcium	Iron
Breakfast						
Subtotal	___	___	___	___	___	___
Snack						
Subtotal	___	___	___	___	___	___
Lunch						
Subtotal	___	___	___	___	___	___
Snack						
Subtotal	___	___	___	___	___	___
Dinner						
Subtotal	___	___	___	___	___	___
Snack						
Subtotal	___	___	___	___	___	___
Daily total	___	___	___	___	___	___
Daily Nutrient Goals	2200	60	70	300–400*	1000	10–15**

* You need 600 mcg of folic acid daily, but some of that comes from your prenatal supplement.

** You need 30 mg of iron daily, but some of that comes from your prenatal supplement.

WEEK 30

Appointments:

Date _____ Time _____

Date _____ Time _____

Remember to find out if _____

_____

_____

Goals:

Next week I will _____

_____

❀

Instead of a cooked vegetable at dinner, try sliced fresh tomato, raw carrots, coleslaw, or raw green pepper strips. If you don't like cooked spinach, add some raw spinach to your salad.

❀

WEEK 31

HOW ARE THE TWO OF YOU DOING?

Your baby weighs 3½ pounds and is 18 inches long.

You are wondering if everything is okay because you feel so many unusual sensations. It is normal for parts of your body to ache, puff up, itch, swell, sag, get numb, and feel sore. This is fun!

Is it okay to eat chips made with fat replacers?

We'd recommend going easy on any chips. Large amounts of regular chips, which are high in fat, might aggravate indigestion, and chips made with some fat replacers may also cause indigestion and diarrhea.

We're not suggesting that you can't eat foods made with fat substitutes. In some foods, water, air, sugar, or fruit is used to replace some or all of the fat. Other foods contain specially designed ingredients that can either replace fat or act like fat but not replace all of it.

Remember that it will take 55,000 calories to complete the development of a full-term baby, so it's as important as ever to make good food choices for both of you.

WEEK 31

PREGNANCY FOOD CHECKLIST

Goals:
- 2–3 servings of protein-rich foods
- 3 servings of calcium-rich foods
- 5 or more fruits and vegetables
- 6 or more servings of breads, grains, and cereals

	Calories	Protein	Vit C	Folic Acid	Calcium	Iron
Breakfast						
Subtotal	___	___	___	___	___	___
Snack						
Subtotal	___	___	___	___	___	___
Lunch						
Subtotal	___	___	___	___	___	___
Snack						
Subtotal	___	___	___	___	___	___
Dinner						
Subtotal	___	___	___	___	___	___
Snack						
Subtotal	___	___	___	___	___	___
Daily total	___	___	___	___	___	___
Daily Nutrient Goals	2200	60	70	300–400*	1000	10–15**

* You need 600 mcg of folic acid daily, but some of that comes from your prenatal supplement.

** You need 30 mg of iron daily, but some of that comes from your prenatal supplement.

WEEK 31

Appointments:

Date _____ Time _____

Date _____ Time _____

Remember to find out if _____

_____

_____

Goals:

Next week I will _____

_____

❦

People may try to predict the sex of your baby based on the shape of your belly—high, low, pointy, or big all around. How you carry has to do with your body type, how much room you have between your hips and your chest, or even how your baby is positioned in the uterus. It has nothing to do with your baby's sex.

❦

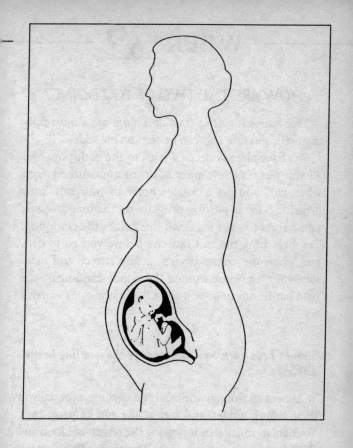

WEEK 32

HOW ARE THE TWO OF YOU DOING?

Your baby's digestive tract and lungs are almost fully matured, and fine hair can be seen on his scalp.

You have already made 4 trips to the bathroom and all you want is a few more hours of undisturbed sleep when *zap!* you get a charley horse in your calf. Your growing baby is putting pressure on the blood vessels and nerves to your legs, and this causes the cramping. Try stretching the calf muscles before you go to bed, and when the cramp occurs, gently stretch and massage your leg. Some women claim that standing on the cold bathroom floor will relax the cramp—it's worth a try.

Should I cut back on salt to reduce the swelling in my ankles?

Almost all women notice a little swelling, especially in their hands, ankles, and feet at the end of pregnancy. Your enlarging uterus is slowing the return of blood and fluid from your arms and legs. Restricting fluids or salt can make the problem worse. Drinking plenty of liquids actually helps keep fluid moving through your body. So does exercise—try taking a daily walk, and elevate your feet when you sit. Tight clothing, snug-fitting rings, and crossing your legs while sitting can make the swelling worse. The good news is that your body will begin to get rid of all this extra fluid as soon as you deliver.

WEEK 32

PREGNANCY FOOD CHECKLIST

Goals:
- 2–3 servings of protein-rich foods
- 3 servings of calcium-rich foods
- 5 or more fruits and vegetables
- 6 or more servings of breads, grains, and cereals

	Calories	Protein	Vit C	Folic Acid	Calcium	Iron
Breakfast						
Subtotal	___	___	___	___	___	___
Snack						
Subtotal	___	___	___	___	___	___
Lunch						
Subtotal	___	___	___	___	___	___
Snack						
Subtotal	___	___	___	___	___	___
Dinner						
Subtotal	___	___	___	___	___	___
Snack						
Subtotal	___	___	___	___	___	___
Daily total	___	___	___	___	___	___
Daily Nutrient Goals	2200	60	70	300–400*	1000	10–15**

* You need 600 mcg of folic acid daily, but some of that comes from your prenatal supplement.

** You need 30 mg of iron daily, but some of that comes from your prenatal supplement.

Appointments:

Date _____ Time _____

Date _____ Time _____

Remember to find out if _____

_____

_____

Goals:

Next week I will _____

_____

My weight is _____

❀

Your health care practitioner may begin seeing you every
two weeks.

❀

WEEK 33

HOW ARE THE TWO OF YOU DOING?

Your baby weighs a little over 4 pounds and is 19 inches long. Her eyes are blue, but they may change color after birth.

You may feel uncomfortable in your own body. Your feet don't fit in your shoes, your fingers are too big for your rings, your breasts are enormous; you even move differently, bumping into furniture and feeling off balance. Carrying a baby for nine months affects every inch of your body, but you'll be pleasantly surprised at how quickly your body bounces back to the old you after delivery.

Can I do anything to relieve my heartburn?

Within the next few weeks, your baby will drop lower into the birth canal, and that will help. In the meantime, don't eat late at night or lie down or recline after eating. Elevating the head of your bed or sleeping on two pillows may help.

Heartburn has nothing to do with your heart. It happens when the circular muscle between your stomach and food tube (esophagus) relaxes and opens. The acidic stomach contents splash back onto the delicate tissues in your food tube, causing burning and burping. Coffee, chocolate, alcohol, peppermint, spearmint, smoking, and high fat foods tend to relax this muscle. If you end a meal with cheesecake you might aggravate heartburn. We don't know why, but nonfat milk seems to tighten the muscle and decrease heartburn. Try ending meals with a small glass (an ounce or two is enough), and drink a little at bedtime. Check with your health care practitioner before you use antacids.

WEEK 33

PREGNANCY FOOD CHECKLIST

Goals:
- 2–3 servings of protein-rich foods
- 3 servings of calcium-rich foods
- 5 or more fruits and vegetables
- 6 or more servings of breads, grains, and cereals

	Calories	Protein	Vit C	Folic Acid	Calcium	Iron
Breakfast						
Subtotal	____	____	____	____	____	____
Snack						
Subtotal	____	____	____	____	____	____
Lunch						
Subtotal	____	____	____	____	____	____
Snack						
Subtotal	____	____	____	____	____	____
Dinner						
Subtotal	____	____	____	____	____	____
Snack						
Subtotal	____	____	____	____	____	____
Daily total	____	____	____	____	____	____
Daily Nutrient Goals	2200	60	70	300–400*	1000	10–15**

* You need 600 mcg of folic acid daily, but some of that comes from your prenatal supplement.
** You need 30 mg of iron daily, but some of that comes from your prenatal supplement.

Appointments:

Date _____ Time _____

Date _____ Time _____

Remember to find out if _____

_____

_____

Goals:

Next week I will _____

_____

❊

Be careful. As your due date nears, you are carrying 6 to 8 pounds of baby, about 2 pounds of placenta, up to a quart of amniotic fluid, and your uterus out in front of you. This can throw off your balance.

❊

WEEK 34

HOW ARE THE TWO OF YOU DOING?

Your baby weighs almost 5 pounds.

You may feel your uterus rhythmically contract, get hard, and then relax. Don't panic—this is not labor. These are Braxton-Hicks contractions, named for the obstetrician who first described them. They occur randomly and help tone up your uterus for the real thing.

> Labor pains or contractions occur at regular intervals. As labor progresses they get closer together and stronger, and they last longer.

Do I need to keep taking my prenatal vitamins?

During the last few weeks of pregnancy your baby is growing faster than ever before, and his need for key nutrients is greater than ever. It's smart to keep taking your vitamins. Many health care practitioners will recommend them if you breastfeed. And it's always important to eat well!

PREGNANCY FOOD CHECKLIST

Goals:
- 2–3 servings of protein-rich foods
- 3 servings of calcium-rich foods
- 5 or more fruits and vegetables
- 6 or more servings of breads, grains, and cereals

	Calories	Protein	Vit C	Folic Acid	Calcium	Iron
Breakfast						
Subtotal	____	____	____	____	____	____
Snack						
Subtotal	____	____	____	____	____	____
Lunch						
Subtotal	____	____	____	____	____	____
Snack						
Subtotal	____	____	____	____	____	____
Dinner						
Subtotal	____	____	____	____	____	____
Snack						
Subtotal	____	____	____	____	____	____
Daily total	____	____	____	____	____	____
Daily Nutrient Goals	2200	60	70	300–400*	1000	10–15**

* You need 600 mcg of folic acid daily, but some of that comes from your prenatal supplement.
** You need 30 mg of iron daily, but some of that comes from your prenatal supplement.

WEEK 34

Appointments:

Date _____ Time _____

Date _____ Time _____

Remember to find out if _____

_____

_____

Goals:

Next week I will _____

_____

Though vitamins and minerals are needed for your baby to develop, too much of a good thing can be dangerous. Don't take large doses of any nutrients during pregnancy. Check with your health care practitioner if you are taking more than recommended.

WEEK 35

HOW ARE THE TWO OF YOU DOING?

Your baby weighs 5½ pounds and is 20 inches long. His fine, downy body hair is disappearing.

You may find it easier to breathe and have less indigestion. That's because of "lightening," a shift in your baby's position downward into the birth canal, relieving some of the pressure on your upper body. The bad news is that now he's pressing on your hips, bladder, and rectum.

As I get closer to my due date co-workers and friends often take me out to eat. How can I avoid winding up as big as a house?

Enjoy your last few weeks. Let people fuss over you and take you out. Eating out doesn't have to equal eating poorly or too much.

- Instead of an appetizer and a main course, order two appetizers.
- Start with soup. It takes time to eat, is low to moderate in calories (stay away from cream soups and bisques) and can be loaded with good-for-you vegetables.

- Drink water. It will help fill you up.
- Order salad dressing and gravy on the side or skip them altogether.
- Stick with broiled, baked, or grilled selections rather than fried, battered, or breaded.
- Share dessert with a friend.
- Instead of stuffing yourself, take the leftovers home.

WEEK 35

PREGNANCY FOOD CHECKLIST

Goals:
- 2–3 servings of protein-rich foods
- 3 servings of calcium-rich foods
- 5 or more fruits and vegetables
- 6 or more servings of breads, grains, and cereals

	Calories	Protein	Vit C	Folic Acid	Calcium	Iron
Breakfast						
Subtotal	____	____	____	____	____	____
Snack						
Subtotal	____	____	____	____	____	____
Lunch						
Subtotal	____	____	____	____	____	____
Snack						
Subtotal	____	____	____	____	____	____
Dinner						
Subtotal	____	____	____	____	____	____
Snack						
Subtotal	____	____	____	____	____	____
Daily total	____	____	____	____	____	____
Daily Nutrient Goals	2200	60	70	300–400*	1000	10–15**

* You need 600 mcg of folic acid daily, but some of that comes from your prenatal supplement.

** You need 30 mg of iron daily, but some of that comes from your prenatal supplement.

WEEK 35

Appointments:

Date _____ Time _____

Date _____ Time _____

Remember to find out if _____

_____

_____

Goals:

Next week I will _____

_____

❀

As you carry your baby lower you may feel some numbness or a pins-and-needles sensation in your hip area. Lying on your side can help.

❀

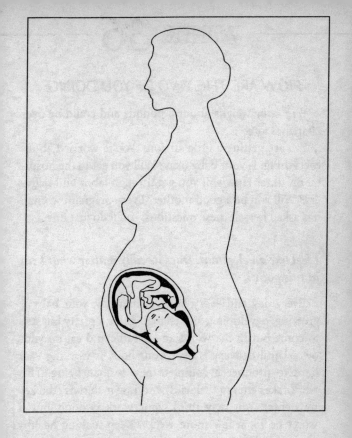

WEEK 36

HOW ARE THE TWO OF YOU DOING?

Your baby weighs about 6 pounds and could be over 20 inches long.

You are getting a little anxious. You're worried about everything: Is your baby okay? Will you get to the hospital on time? How will you get through labor and delivery? Will you be a good mother? Every pregnant woman has asked herself these questions. You'll do just fine.

I feel like an elephant. Does it really matter what I eat at this point?

Every day and every hour in that day, your baby is growing, developing, and changing. It's a pretty big step to come out in the world and breathe and eat on your own. Until delivery is over, your body is working very hard to produce a complete new human being. This work takes energy (calories) and raw materials (the key nutrients). You may think your work is done, but it won't be for a few more weeks. Keep making healthy choices and take good care of both of you.

WEEK 36

PREGNANCY FOOD CHECKLIST

Goals:
- 2–3 servings of protein-rich foods
- 3 servings of calcium-rich foods
- 5 or more fruits and vegetables
- 6 or more servings of breads, grains, and cereals

	Calories	Protein	Vit C	Folic Acid	Calcium	Iron
Breakfast						
Subtotal	____	____	____	____	____	____
Snack						
Subtotal	____	____	____	____	____	____
Lunch						
Subtotal	____	____	____	____	____	____
Snack						
Subtotal	____	____	____	____	____	____
Dinner						
Subtotal	____	____	____	____	____	____
Snack						
Subtotal	____	____	____	____	____	____
Daily total	____	____	____	____	____	____
Daily Nutrient Goals	2200	60	70	300–400*	1000	10–15**

* You need 600 mcg of folic acid daily, but some of that comes from your prenatal supplement.
** You need 30 mg of iron daily, but some of that comes from your prenatal supplement.

WEEK 36

Appointments:

Date _____ Time _____

Date _____ Time _____

Remember to find out if _____

_____

_____

Goals:

Next week I will _____

_____

My weight is _____

❀

Your health care practitioner may ask you to come in weekly for the rest of your pregnancy.

❀

WEEK 37

HOW ARE THE TWO OF YOU DOING?

Your baby weighs almost 6½ pounds, and she is facing downward, waiting to make her grand appearance.

You may notice that your baby isn't moving too much. Don't worry. There's simply not enough room for her to do much more than wiggle and stretch.

Is it true that you shouldn't fast at the end of pregnancy?

Research has shown that when pregnant women fast for as little as a day, they increase their chance of early labor. Fasting offers no health benefits. Most pregnant women are not encouraged to observe religious fast days at this point, either.

WEEK 37

PREGNANCY FOOD CHECKLIST

Goals:
- 2–3 servings of protein-rich foods
- 3 servings of calcium-rich foods
- 5 or more fruits and vegetables
- 6 or more servings of breads, grains, and cereals

	Calories	Protein	Vit C	Folic Acid	Calcium	Iron
Breakfast						
Subtotal	____	____	____	____	____	____
Snack						
Subtotal	____	____	____	____	____	____
Lunch						
Subtotal	____	____	____	____	____	____
Snack						
Subtotal	____	____	____	____	____	____
Dinner						
Subtotal	____	____	____	____	____	____
Snack						
Subtotal	____	____	____	____	____	____
Daily total	____	____	____	____	____	____
Daily Nutrient Goals	2200	60	70	300–400*	1000	10–15**

* You need 600 mcg of folic acid daily, but some of that comes from your prenatal supplement.

** You need 30 mg of iron daily, but some of that comes from your prenatal supplement.

— week 37 —

Appointments:

Date _____ Time _____

Date _____ Time _____

Remember to find out if _____

_____

_____

Goals:

Next week I will _____

_____

My weight is _____

You may have mood swings that surprise even you. These emotional changes are common at the end of pregnancy. Simply being aware that this may happen will make it easier to deal with.

WEEK 38

HOW ARE THE TWO OF YOU DOING?

Your baby weighs close to 7 pounds and may be 21 inches long. He's getting rounder and plumper with each passing day.

You are impatient to have labor start.

HOW FAR ALONG ARE YOU?

Effacement: The softening and thinning of the cervix that occurs during labor, or sometimes before labor starts. Effacement is reported as 0% to 100%.

Dilation: The size of the opening of the cervix, measured from 0 to 10 centimeters. Ten is completely open, and this occurs shortly before delivery.

Station: How far your baby has dropped into the birth canal. Zero is your spine, minus numbers are for positions above this; plus numbers for stations below.

Keep making good food choices for both of you. You need extra energy to see you through the last sprint before delivery. You are working very hard!

PREGNANCY FOOD CHECKLIST

Goals:
- 2–3 servings of protein-rich foods
- 3 servings of calcium-rich foods
- 5 or more fruits and vegetables
- 6 or more servings of breads, grains, and cereals

	Calories	Protein	Vit C	Folic Acid	Calcium	Iron
Breakfast						
Subtotal	____	____	____	____	____	____
Snack						
Subtotal	____	____	____	____	____	____
Lunch						
Subtotal	____	____	____	____	____	____
Snack						
Subtotal	____	____	____	____	____	____
Dinner						
Subtotal	____	____	____	____	____	____
Snack						
Subtotal	____	____	____	____	____	____
Daily total	____	____	____	____	____	____
Daily Nutrient Goals	2200	60	70	300–400*	1000	10–15**

* You need 600 mcg of folic acid daily, but some of that comes from your prenatal supplement.
** You need 30 mg of iron daily, but some of that comes from your prenatal supplement.

WEEK 38

Appointments:

Date _____ Time _____

Date _____ Time _____

Remember to find out if _____

_____

_____

Goals:

Next week I will _____

_____

My weight is _____

Women typically gain 7 to 11 pounds of fat during pregnancy. These stores of energy and nutrient reserves are used during labor and delivery, and they help support breastfeeding. This is nature's way of making sure you are not caught short.

WEEK 39

HOW ARE THE TWO OF YOU DOING?

Your baby weighs a little over 7 pounds and is completely developed and ready to be on her own. She just needs to accumulate a little more fat.

You have had it! At this point most women vow never to be pregnant again. Luckily, most of us forget this vow once we see our baby.

How will I feed my baby?

As delivery draws near, you worry less about what you are eating and more about how you will feed your baby. Your health care practitioner will help you take each step along the way. A lactation consultant may be available in the hospital.

We'd encourage you to consider breastfeeding. Very few mothers decide to nurse or use formula without worrying whether their choice is the right one. Take time to learn about both. This, like many things you'll decide for your baby, has no right or wrong answer. You and your partner will make the best decisions for your family.

WEEK 39

PREGNANCY FOOD CHECKLIST

Goals:
- 2–3 servings of protein-rich foods
- 3 servings of calcium-rich foods
- 5 or more fruits and vegetables
- 6 or more servings of breads, grains, and cereals

	Calories	Protein	Vit C	Folic Acid	Calcium	Iron
Breakfast						
Subtotal	____	____	____	____	____	____
Snack						
Subtotal	____	____	____	____	____	____
Lunch						
Subtotal	____	____	____	____	____	____
Snack						
Subtotal	____	____	____	____	____	____
Dinner						
Subtotal	____	____	____	____	____	____
Snack						
Subtotal	____	____	____	____	____	____
Daily total	____	____	____	____	____	____
Daily Nutrient Goals	2200	60	70	300–400*	1000	10–15**

* You need 600 mcg of folic acid daily, but some of that comes from your prenatal supplement.

** You need 30 mg of iron daily, but some of that comes from your prenatal supplement.

WEEK 39

Appointments:

Date _____ Time _____

Date _____ Time _____

Remember to find out if _____

_____

_____

Goals:

Next week I will _____

_____

My weight is _____

❊

If you think your water has broken, call your health care practitioner. This is actually a crack in the amniotic sac allowing some fluid to escape. You may experience a gush of clear fluid (at least a cup) or a continual leaking. It's a sign that labor is not far off.

❊

WEEK 40

HOW ARE THE TWO OF YOU DOING?

Your baby is as big as he is going to get, about 7½ pounds and 21 inches.

You are counting the days till your due date but remember that only 1 woman in 20 delivers on her actual due date. The rest deliver anywhere from 2 weeks before till 2 weeks after the calculated date.

Should I eat or drink anything if I think I'm in labor?

Most health care practitioners recommend not eating if you are in labor. This is a precaution in case you get anesthesia. It is usually all right to drink water, suck on ice chips or ice pops, or even sip clear fluids like fruit juice. Your childbirth instructor may have suggested sucking on lollipops during labor.

GIVE SOME THOUGHT TO THE FUTURE:

You've spent the last nine months practicing good health habits, and you've learned a lot about how to eat well. Now it's your turn to pass on these good habits to your new baby.

How you take care of your family now will affect their health 20 years from now. Take good care of all of you.

WEEK 40

PREGNANCY FOOD CHECKLIST

Goals:
- 2–3 servings of protein-rich foods
- 3 servings of calcium-rich foods
- 5 or more fruits and vegetables
- 6 or more servings of breads, grains, and cereals

	Calories	Protein	Vit C	Folic Acid	Calcium	Iron
Breakfast						
Subtotal	____	____	____	____	____	____
Snack						
Subtotal	____	____	____	____	____	____
Lunch						
Subtotal	____	____	____	____	____	____
Snack						
Subtotal	____	____	____	____	____	____
Dinner						
Subtotal	____	____	____	____	____	____
Snack						
Subtotal	____	____	____	____	____	____
Daily total	____	____	____	____	____	____
Daily Nutrient Goals	2200	60	70	300–400*	1000	10–15**

* You need 600 mcg of folic acid daily, but some of that comes from your prenatal supplement.

** You need 30 mg of iron daily, but some of that comes from your prenatal supplement.

WEEK 40

Appointments:

Date _____ Time _____

Date _____ Time _____

Remember to find out if _____

_____

_____

Goals:

Next week I will _____

_____

My weight is _____

My baby's weight is _____

Nothing can compare to the miracle of your baby's birth. Congratulations! You did a great job taking care of your little one, and we know you'll do a great job from here on.

PART II

FOOD VALUES

All protein values are given in grams.

All vitamin C, calcium, and iron values are given in milligrams.

All folic acid values are given in micrograms.

A dash (—) indicates data not available.

If you'd like a bigger reference with more than 21,000 food values listed, look for *The Most Complete Food Counter*, also available from Pocket Books.

Food	Portion	Calories	Protein	Vit C	Folic Acid	Calcium	Iron
ALFALFA							
Sprouts	1 tbsp	1	tr	tr	1	1	tr
ALMONDS							
Oil Roasted Salted	1 oz	174	5	tr	18	55	2
APPLE							
Applesauce	1/2 cup	97	tr	2	1	5	tr
Fresh	1	81	tr	8	4	10	tr
Juice	1cup	116	tr	2	tr	16	1
APRICOTS							
Dried Halves	5	42	1	1	2	8	1
Fresh	3	51	1	11	9	15	1
Nectar	1 cup	141	1	1	3	17	1
ARTICHOKE							
Fresh	1 med (4 oz)	60	4	12	61	54	2
Hearts Cooked	1/2 cup	42	3	8	42	38	1
ARUGULA							
Raw	1/2 cup	2	tr	—	10	16	—
ASPARAGUS							
Cooked	4 spears	14	2	7	88	12	tr
AVOCADO							
Fresh	1	324	4	16	124	22	2
BACON							
Fried	3 strips	109	6	0	1	2	tr

Food	Portion	Calories	Protein	Vit C	Folic Acid	Calcium	Iron
Substitute Cooked	1 strip	25	1	0	4	2	tr
BAGEL							
Plain Toasted	1 (3 1/2 in)	195	8	0	11	53	3
BANANA							
Fresh	1	105	1	10	22	7	tr
BEANS							
Baked Beans	1/2 cup	118	6	—	30	64	tr
Baked Beans w/ Franks	1/2 cup	182	9	3	38	62	2
Refried Beans	1/2 cup	43	2	0	9	9	1
Sprouts	1/2 cup	8	1	tr	6	9	tr
Three Bean Salad	3/4 cup	230	5	3	5	58	3
BEEF							
Beef Stew	1 cup	179	10	—	13	34	2
Bottom Round Braised	3 oz	241	24	0	8	5	3
Brisket Braised	3 oz	183	26	0	7	5	2
Chopped Beef Steak Fried	1 serv (4 oz)	311	22	0	6	12	3
Chuck Roast Braised	3 oz	293	23	0	5	11	3
Eye Round Roasted	3 oz	153	24	0	6	4	2
Filet Mignon Broiled	3 oz	270	21	0	5	7	3
Flank Steak Braised	3 oz	224	23	0	7	6	3
Ground Extra Lean Broiled	3 oz	217	22	0	8	6	2
Ground Regular Broiled	3 oz	246	20	0	8	9	2

Food	Portion	Calories	Protein	Vit C	Folic Acid	Calcium	Iron
Hamburger Helper							
Meat Loaf as prep	1/6 loaf	270	24	0	16	40	3
Porterhouse Steak Broiled	3 oz	260	21	0	6	7	2
Rib Steak Broiled	3 oz	261	21	0	6	11	2
Shepherds Pie	1 serv (7 oz)	282	16	4	20	120	3
Shortribs Braised	3 oz	400	18	—	4	10	2
Stroganoff	3/4 cup	260	14	3	12	60	2
Swiss Steak	4.6 oz	214	23	14	9	17	3
T-Bone Steak Broiled	3 oz	253	21	0	6	7	2
Top Round Broiled	3 oz	190	26	0	10	6	2
BEEFALO							
Roasted	3 oz	160	26	8	15	21	3
BEETS							
Sliced Cooked	1/2 cup (3 oz)	38	1	3	68	14	1
BISCUIT							
Plain	1 (2 oz)	212	4	tr	7	141	2
W/Egg	1 (4.8 oz)	316	11	0	61	154	3
W/Egg & Bacon	1 (5.2 oz)	458	17	3	60	189	4
W/Egg & Ham	1 (6.7 oz)	442	20	0	65	221	5
W/Sausage	1 (4.4 oz)	485	12	tr	46	128	3
BLACK BEANS							
Cooked	1 cup	227	15	0	256	47	4

159

Food	Portion	Calories	Protein	Vit C	Folic Acid	Calcium	Iron
BLACKEYE PEAS							
Cooked	1 cup	198	13	1	356	42	4
BLUEBERRIES							
Fresh	1 cup	82	1	19	9	9	tr
BLUEFISH							
Fresh Baked	3 oz	135	22	tr	2	8	1
BRAN							
Kretschmer							
Toasted Wheat Bran	1/3 cup	57	6	0	49	26	4
Quacker Oat Bran	1/2 cup (1.4 oz)	150	7	—	8	20	3
BRAZIL NUTS							
Dried	1 oz	186	4	tr	1	50	1
BREAD							
Banana	1 slice (2 oz)	195	3	1	7	13	1
Challah Egg Bread	1 slice (1.4 oz)	115	4	0	28	37	1
Corn Sticks	1 (2 oz)	165	3	0	4	63	tr
Focaccia Rosemary	1 piece (3.5 oz)	251	6	tr	38	13	3
French	1 slice (1 oz)	78	3	0	9	21	1
Irish Soda Bread	1 slice (2 oz)	174	4	1	6	49	2
Italian	1 slice (1 oz)	81	3	0	9	23	1
Pita	1 reg (2 oz)	165	5	0	14	52	2
Raisin	1 slice	71	2	—	9	17	1

Food	Portion	Calories	Protein	Vit C	Folic Acid	Calcium	Iron
Rye	1 slice	83	3	—	16	23	1
Seven Grain	1 slice	65	3	tr	12	24	1
Sourdough	1 slice (1 oz)	78	3	0	9	21	1
Texas Toast	1 serv (15.5 oz)	1088	35	0	454	91	5
White Toasted	1 slice	67	2	0	6	27	1
Whole Wheat	1 slice	70	3	—	14	20	1
BREAKFAST BAR							
Nutri-Grain Strawberry	1 (1.3 oz)	140	2	0	100	300	2
BREAKFAST DRINKS							
Pillsbury Instant Breakfast Chocolate as prep w/milk	1 serv	290	14	18	100	250	5
Pillsbury Instant Breakfast Vanilla as prep w/milk	1 serv	300	14	18	100	250	5
BROCCOLI							
Spears Cooked	1/2 cup	25	3	37	28	127	1
BROWNIE							
Plain	1, 2 in sq (2.1 oz)	243	3	3	17	25	1
BRUSSELS SPROUTS							
Cooked	1/2 cup	30	2	48	47	28	1
BUCKWHEAT							
Groats Cooked	1 cup (5.9 oz)	647	6	0	24	12	1

Food	Portion	Calories	Protein	Vit C	Folic Acid	Calcium	Iron
BULGUR							
Cooked	1 cup (6.3 oz)	151	7	0	33	18	2
BUTTER							
Stick	1 pat (5 g)	36	tr	0	tr	1	tr
Whipped	1 pat (4 g)	27	tr	—	tr	1	tr
CABBAGE							
Green Raw Shredded	1/2 cup (1.2 oz)	9	1	11	15	17	tr
Green Shredded Cooked	1/2 cup (2.6 oz)	17	1	15	15	23	tr
Red Raw Shredded	1/2 cup	10	tr	20	7	18	tr
Red Shredded Cooked	1/2 cup	16	1	26	9	28	tr
Stuffed Cabbage	1 (6 oz)	373	25	7	22	339	3
CAKE							
Angelfood	1/12 cake (1.9 oz)	142	4	0	2	3	tr
Carrot w/ Icing	1/12 cake (3.9 oz)	484	5	1	14	27	1
Cheesecake	1/6 cake (2.8 oz)	256	4	—	12	50	1
Coffeecake Crumb Topped	1/12 cake (2.1 oz)	240	4	tr	9	67	1
Eclair	1 (3 oz)	262	6	tr	14	63	1
Kellogg's Pop-Tarts Apple Cinnamon	1 (1.8 oz)	210	2	0	40	0	2
Kellogg's Pop-Tarts Low Fat Strawberry	1 (1.8 oz)	190	2	0	40	0	2

Food	Portion	Calories	Protein	Vit C	Folic Acid	Calcium	Iron
Kellogg's Pop-Tarts							
Strawberry	1 (1.8 oz)	200	2	0	40	0	2
Pound Fat Free	1 cake (12 oz)	961	18	1	14	146	7
Tiramisu	1 piece (5.1 oz)	409	7	1	16	114	1
CANADIAN BACON							
Grilled	1 pkg (6 oz)	257	34	0	6	14	1
CANDY							
Butterscotch	1 piece (6 g)	24	0	0	0	0	0
Caramels	1 piece (8 g)	31	tr	—	0	11	tr
Carob Bar	1 (3.1 oz)	453	11	—	27	391	
Fudge Chocolate	1 piece (0.6 oz)	65	tr	0	0	7	tr
Milk Chocolate	1 bar (1.55 oz)	226	3	tr	4	84	1
CANTALOUPE							
Fresh	1/2	94	2	113	46	28	1
CARROTS							
Juice	6 oz	73	2	16	7	44	1
Raw	1 (2.5 oz)	31	1	7	10	19	tr
CASHEWS							
Cashew Butter	1 tbsp	94	3	0	11	7	1
Dry Roasted Salted	1 oz	163	4	0	20	13	2
CAULIFLOWER							
Cooked	1/2 cup (2.2 oz)	14	1	28	27	10	tr

Food	Portion	Calories	Protein	Vit C	Folic Acid	Calcium	Iron
Flowerets Raw	3 (2 oz)	14	1	26	32	12	tr
CELERY							
Raw	1 stalk (1.3 oz)	6	tr	3	11	16	tr
CEREAL							
100% Bran	1/3 cup (1 oz)	80	4	0	100	20	8
All-Bran	1/2 cup (1.1 oz)	80	4	15	100	150	5
Cap'n Crunch	3/4 cup	113	2	0	157	6	5
Cheerios	1 cup (1 oz)	110	3	15	100	40	8
Cinnamon Toast Crunch	3/4 cup (1 oz)	130	1	15	100	40	5
Cocoa Puffs	1 cup (1 oz)	120	1	15	100	20	5
Corn Chex	1 cup (1 oz)	110	2	6	100	0	9
Corn Grits Yellow Or White							
Regular & Quick as prep	3/4 cup (6.4 oz)	109	3	0	56	0	1
Farina as prep	3/4 cup (6.1 oz)	88	2	0	40	4	1
Fiber One	1/2 cup (1 oz)	60	2	0	100	40	5
Froot Loops	1 cup (1.1 oz)	120	2	15	100	0	5
Frosted Flakes	3/4 cup (1.1 oz)	120	1	15	100	0	4
Grape-Nuts	1/2 cup (2 oz)	200	6	0	100	20	8
Honey Bunches Of Oats	3/4 cup (1 oz)	120	2	0	100	0	3
Kix	1 1/3 cup (1 oz)	120	2	15	100	40	8
Lucky Charms	1 cup (1 oz)	120	2	15	100	20	5
Oatmeal Instant as prep	1 cup (8.2 oz)	138	6	0	199	215	8

Food	Portion	Calories	Protein	Vit C	Folic Acid	Calcium	Iron
Product 19	1 cup (1 oz)	100	2	60	400	0	18
Puffed Rice	1 cup (0.5 oz)	56	1	0	3	1	4
Rice Krispies	1 1/4 cup (1.2 oz)	120	2	15	100	0	2
Shredded Mini Wheats	1 cup (1.1 oz)	107	3	0	14	11	1
Special K	1 cup (1.1 oz)	110	6	15	140	0	9
Waffle Crisp	1 cup (1 oz)	130	2	0	100	0	2
Wheaties	1 cup (1 oz)	110	3	15	100	0	8
CEREAL BARS							
Golden Grahams Treats							
Chocolate Chunk	1 bar (0.8 oz)	90	1	6	40	—	2
Nutri-Grain							
Apple Cinnamon	1 (1.3 oz)	140	2	0	40	20	2
Rice Krispies Treats	1 (0.8 oz)	90	1	0	20	0	tr
CHEESE							
American Cheese	1 oz	82	5	0	2	159	tr
Blue	1 oz	100	6	0	10	150	tr
Cheddar	1 oz	114	7	0	5	204	tr
Cheddar Lowfat	1 oz	49	9	0	3	118	tr
Fondue	1/2 cup (3.8 oz)	247	15	0	5	514	tr
Mozzarella Part Skim	1 oz	72	7	0	2	183	tr
Muenster	1 oz	104	7	0	3	203	tr
Parmesan Grated	1 tbsp (5 g)	23	2	0	tr	69	tr

Food	Portion	Calories	Protein	Vit C	Folic Acid	Calcium	Iron
Provolone	1 oz	100	7	0	3	214	tr
Souffle	1 serv (7 oz)	504	23	tr	38	446	2
Swiss	1 oz	107	8	0	2	272	tr
CHERRIES							
Fresh	10	49	1	5	3	10	tr
CHESTNUTS							
Roasted	2 to 3 (1 oz)	70	1	7	10	8	tr
CHICKEN							
Boneless Breaded & Fried w/ Barbecue Sauce	6 pieces (4.6 oz)	330	17	tr	28	21	1
Breast Batter Dipped & Fried	1/2 breast (4.9 oz)	364	35	0	8	28	1
Breast w/ Skin Roasted	1/2 breast (3.4 oz)	193	29	0	3	14	1
Breast w/o Skin Roasted	1/2 breast (3 oz)	142	27	0	3	13	1
Broiler/Fryer w/ Skin Roasted	1/2 chicken (10.5 oz)	715	82	0	16	45	4
Chicken & Dumplings	3/4 cup	256	23	4	10	61	2
Chicken Cacciatore	3/4 cup	394	33	40	18	45	4
Chicken Teriyaki	1 serv (4 oz)	445	45	3	6	37	2
Cornish Hen w/ Skin Roasted	1/2 hen (4 oz)	296	25	1	3	15	1

Food	Portion	Calories	Protein	Vit C	Folic Acid	Calcium	Iron
Drumstick w/ Skin							
Batter Dipped & Fried	1 (2.6 oz)	193	16	0	6	12	1
Drumstick w/ Skin Roasted	1 (1.8 oz)	112	14	0	4	6	1
Wing w/ Skin							
Batter Dipped & Fried	1 (1.7 oz)	159	10	0	3	10	1
Wing w/ Skin Roasted	1 (1.2 oz)	99	9	0	1	5	tr
CHICKPEAS							
Cooked	1 cup	269	15	2	282	80	5
CHICORY							
Raw	1/2 cup (1.6 oz)	8	tr	1	17	9	tr
CHILI							
Con Carne w/ Beans	8.9 oz	254	25	2	30	67	5
CHIPS							
Corn	1 oz	153	2	0	6	36	tr
Potato	1 oz	152	2	9	13	7	tr
Potato Sticks	1/2 cup (0.6 oz)	94	1	9	7	3	tr
Tortilla Nacho	1 oz	141	2	1	4	42	tr
CHOCOLATE							
Chips Semisweet	60 pieces (1 oz)	136	1	0	1	9	1
Syrup	2 tbsp	82	1	tr	2	5	1
CLAMS							
Meat Only	1 cup	236	41	—	158	148	45

Food	Portion	Calories	Protein	Vit C	Folic Acid	Calcium	Iron
COCOA							
Hot Cocoa	1 cup	218	9	2	12	298	1
COCONUT							
Fresh	1 piece (1.5 oz)	159	2	2	12	6	1
COFFEE							
Cappuccino	1 cup (8 fl oz)	77	4	1	6	148	tr
Coffee Con Leche	1 cup (8 fl oz)	77	4	1	6	148	tr
Decaffeinated	6 oz	4	tr	0	0	6	tr
Espresso	1 cup (3 fl oz)	2	tr	0	tr	2	tr
Latte w/ Skim Milk	13 oz	88	8	2	13	304	tr
Latte w/ Whole Milk	13 oz	152	8	2	12	293	tr
Regular	6 oz	4	tr	0	0	6	tr
Whitener Powder							
Nondairy	1 tsp	11	tr	0	0	tr	tr
COLLARDS							
Cooked	1/2 cup	17	1	8	4	15	tr
COOKIES							
Animal	11 crackers (1 oz)	126	2	0	4	12	1
Chocolate Chip	1 (0.4 oz)	48	1	0	1	2	tr
Chocolate w/ Creme Filling	1 (0.35 oz)	47	1	0	0	3	tr
Fig Newtons	1 (0.56 oz)	56	1	—	2	10	tr
Fortune	1 (0.28 oz)	30	tr	0	1	1	tr

168

Food	Portion	Calories	Protein	Vit C	Folic Acid	Calcium	Iron
Graham	1 squares (0.24 oz)	30	1	0	1	3	tr
Peanut Butter	1 (0.5 oz)	69	1	0	1	2	tr
Vanilla Sandwich	1 (0.35 oz)	48	tr	0	0	3	tr
CORN							
Cooked	1/2 cup	67	2	2	19	2	tr
Cream Style	1/2 cup	93	2	6	57	4	tr
Fritters	1 (1 oz)	62	2	1	3	21	tr
On-The-Cob	1 ear (2.2 oz)	59	2	3	19	2	tr
COTTAGE CHEESE							
Creamed	1 cup (7.4 oz)	217	26	tr	26	126	tr
Lowfat 1%	1 cup (7.9 oz)	164	28	tr	28	138	tr
Pot Cheese	1 cup (5.1 oz)	123	25	0	21	46	tr
COUSCOUS							
Cooked	1 cup (5.5 oz)	176	6	0	24	13	1
CRAB							
Baked	1 (3.8 oz)	160	29	3	20	415	1
Cake	1 (2 oz)	160	11	tr	10	202	1
Soft-Shell Fried	1 (4.4 oz)	334	11	tr	20	55	2
CRACKERS							
Cheese	14 (1/2 oz)	71	1	0	4	21	1
Melba Toast	1 (5 g)	19	1	0	1	5	tr
Oyster Cracker	1 (1 g)	4	tr	0	tr	1	tr

169

Food	Portion	Calories	Protein	Vit C	Folic Acid	Calcium	Iron
Saltines	1 (3 g)	13	tr	0	1	4	tr
Whole Wheat	1 (4 g)	18	tr	0	1	2	tr
CRANBERRY							
Juice Cocktail	1 cup	147	tr	108	1	8	tr
Sauce	1/4 cup	105	tr	2	—	3	tr
CREAM							
Light Coffee	1 tbsp (0.5 oz)	29	tr	tr	tr	14	tr
Whipped	1 cup (4.1 oz)	411	5	1	9	77	tr
CREAM CHEESE							
Plain	1 oz	99	2	0	4	23	tr
CROISSANT							
Plain	1 (2 oz)	232	5	—	16	21	1
W/ Egg & Cheese	1 (4.5 oz)	368	13	tr	47	244	2
CUCUMBER							
Fresh	1 (11 oz)	38	2	16	38	43	1
Kimchee	1/2 cup (1.8 oz)	36	tr	6	6	10	tr
CUSTARD							
Baked	1/2 cup (5 oz)	148	7	1	44	158	tr
DANISH PASTRY							
Cheese	1 (3.2 oz)	353	6	3	55	70	2
Fruit	1 (3.3 oz)	335	5	2	31	22	1

Food	Portion	Calories	Protein	Vit C	Folic Acid	Calcium	Iron
DATES							
Whole Dried	5	224	1	0	5	24	1
DELI MEATS/COLD CUTS							
Bologna Beef	1 oz	88	4	6	1	3	tr
Liverwurst Pork	1 oz	92	4	—	9	7	2
Salami Cooked	1 oz	71	4	3	1	4	1
DOUGHNUTS							
Glazed	1 (2.1 oz)	242	4	—	13	26	1
DUCK							
W/ Skin Roasted	1 cup (4.9 oz)	472	27	0	8	15	4
EGG							
Deviled	2 halves	145	6	0	25	31	1
Hard Cooked	1	77	6	0	22	25	1
Omelette Plain	1 serv (3.5 oz)	172	15	0	30	63	2
Salad	1/2 cup	307	13	0	49	189	2
Scrambled Plain	2 (3.3 oz)	199	13	3	53	54	2
Sunny Side Up	1	91	6	0	18	25	1
EGGNOG							
Eggnog	1 cup	342	10	4	2	330	1
EGGPLANT							
Cooked	1/2 cup	13	tr	1	7	3	tr

Food	Portion	Calories	Protein	Vit C	Folic Acid	Calcium	Iron
ENDIVE							
Chopped	1/2 cup	4	tr	2	36	13	tr
ENGLISH MUFFIN							
W/ Butter	1 (2.2 oz)	189	5	1	57	103	2
w/ Egg Cheese & Sausage	1 (5.8 oz)	487	22	2	54	196	3
FIGS							
Dried	5	244	3	1	7	235	2
FISH							
Gefilte Fish	1 piece (1.5 oz)	35	4	—	1	10	1
Sticks	1 stick (1 oz)	76	4	—	5	6	tr
FRENCH TOAST							
Sticks	5 (4.9 oz)	513	8	0	82	78	3
W/Butter	2 slices (4.7 oz)	356	10	tr	73	73	2
FRUIT							
Fruit Punch	6 fl oz	87	tr	55	2	14	tr
Fruit Salad	1 serv (6 oz)	59	1	58	15	18	tr
Tropicana Tangerine							
Orange Juice	8 fl oz	110	2	72	60	20	0
GELATIN							
All Flavors	1 serv (4.75 oz)	128	2	0	0	6	0
Low Calorie	1/2 cup	8	2	0	0	tr	tr

Food	Portion	Calories	Protein	Vit C	Folic Acid	Calcium	Iron
GOAT							
Roasted	3 oz	122	23	—	5	15	3
GOOSE							
W/Skin Roasted	6.6 oz	574	47	0	4	25	5
GRANOLA							
Bar Chewy							
Chocolate Coated							
Chocolate Chip	1 (1 oz)	132	2	0	7	29	1
Bar Chewy							
Peanut Butter	1 (1 oz)	121	3	0	9	26	1
Cereal	1/2 cup (2.1 oz)	285	9	1	53	45	3
Kellogg's Cereal Low Fat	1/2 cup (1.7 oz)	190	4	2	100	20	2
GRAPEFRUIT							
Fresh Samantha Juice	1 cup (8 oz)	101	3	54	8	0	0
Pink	1/2	37	1	47	15	13	tr
Tropicana Juice Ruby Red							
w/Calcium	8 oz	90	1	96	16	402	0
White Sections	1 cup	76	2	77	23	28	tr
GRAPES							
Fresh	10	36	tr	5	2	5	tr
Juice	1 cup	155	1	tr	7	22	1

Food	Portion	Calories	Protein	Vit C	Folic Acid	Calcium	Iron
GREEN BEANS							
Canned	1/2 cup	13	1	3	22	18	1
Italian	1/2 cup	13	1	3	22	18	1
Raw	1/2 cup	17	1	9	20	21	1
HADDOCK							
Breaded & Fried	1 piece (3.5 oz)	187	23	0	3	40	1
HALIBUT							
Baked	5.6 oz	380	29	—	2	6	1
HAM							
Canned Extra Lean Roasted	3 oz	116	18	0	4	5	1
Center Slice Lean Roasted	4 oz	220	31	0	6	11	1
Croquettes	1 (3.1 oz)	217	12	tr	11	50	2
Patty Cooked	1 patty (2 oz)	203	8	0	2	5	1
Salad	1/2 cup	287	16	1	22	33	2
Sliced Extra Lean	1 oz	37	5	7	1	2	tr
HAMBURGER							
Double Patty w/Bun	1 reg	544	30	0	38	87	5
Double Patty w/Cheese & Bun	1 reg	457	28	0	29	232	3
Single Patty w/Bun	1 reg	275	12	0	25	63	2
Single Patty w/Cheese & Bun	1 reg	320	15	0	26	140	2

Food	Portion	Calories	Protein	Vit C	Folic Acid	Calcium	Iron
Triple Patty w/Cheese & Bun	1 lg	769	56	3	51	282	8
HEARTS OF PALM							
Canned	1 (1.2 oz)	9	1	3	13	19	1
HERRING							
Fried	1 serv (3.5 oz)	233	23	0	10	35	1
Pickled	1/2 oz	39	2	—	tr	12	tr
HOMINY							
White	1 cup (5.6 oz)	482	2	0	2	16	1
HONEY							
Honey	1 tbsp (0.7 oz)	64	tr	tr	0	1	tr
HOT DOG							
Corndog	1	460	17	0	60	101	6
W/Bun Chili	1	297	14	3	50	19	3
W/Bun Plain	1	242	10	tr	30	24	2
HUMMUS							
Hummus	1/3 cup	140	4	6	49	41	1
ICE CREAM AND FROZEN DESSERTS							
Dixie Cup Chocolate	1 (3.5 fl oz)	125	2	tr	9	63	1
Dixie Cup Strawberry	1 (3.5 fl oz)	112	2	5	7	70	tr
Dixie Cup Vanilla	1 (3.5 fl oz)	116	2	tr	3	74	tr
Gelato Chocolate Hazelnut	1/2 cup (5.3 oz)	370	9	1	35	179	2

Food	Portion	Calories	Protein	Vit C	Folic Acid	Calcium	Iron
Gelato Vanilla	1/2 cup (3 oz)	211	3	tr	15	67	tr
Sundae Caramel	1 (5.4 oz)	303	7	3	12	189	tr
Sundae Hot Fudge	1 (5.4 oz)	284	6	2	9	207	tr
Vanilla Light	1/2 cup (2.3 oz)	92	3	1	4	92	tr
ICED TEA							
Instant Mix Sweetened							
As Prep	9 oz	87	tr	0	10	6	tr
JAM/JELLY							
Jam	1 tbsp (0.7 oz)	48	tr	2	7	4	tr
Jelly	1 tbsp (0.7 oz)	52	tr	tr	0	2	tr
KALE							
Fresh Cooked	1/2 cup	21	1	27	9	47	1
KETCHUP							
Ketchup	1 tbsp	16	tr	2	2	3	tr
KIDNEY BEANS							
Canned	1 cup	208	13	3	126	69	3
KNISH							
Potato	1 med (3.5 oz)	166	4	4	17	27	1
LAMB							
Cubed Lean Only Broiled	3 oz	158	24	—	19	11	2
Curry	3/4 cup	345	26	3	16	24	3
Leg Of Lamb Roasted	3 oz	219	22	—	17	9	2

Food	Portion	Calories	Protein	Vit C	Folic Acid	Calcium	Iron
Loin Chop Broiled	1 chop (2.3 oz)	201	16	—	12	13	1
Rib Chop Broiled	3 oz	307	19	—	12	16	2
Shank Braised	3 oz	206	24	—	14	17	2
Stew	3/4 cup	124	10	20	37	54	1
LEMONADE							
Mix As Prep	9 fl oz	113	0	34	0	29	tr
LENTILS							
Cooked	1 cup	231	18	3	358	37	7
LETTUCE							
Iceberg	1 leaf	3	tr	1	11	4	tr
Romaine Shredded	1/2 cup	4	tr	7	38	10	tr
LIVER							
Beef Pan-Fried	3 oz	184	23	19	187	9	5
Chicken Stewed	1 cup (5 oz)	219	34	22	1077	20	12
Pate	1 tbsp (13 g)	41	5	0	8	9	1
LOBSTER							
Fresh Cooked	1 cup	142	30	—	16	88	1
MACKEREL							
Baked	6.2 oz	354	45	—	4	52	3
Canned	1 cup	296	44	2	10	458	4
Smoked	3.5 oz	296	19	0	1	20	1

Food	Portion	Calories	Protein	Vit C	Folic Acid	Calcium	Iron
MARGARINE							
Diet	1 tsp	17	0	tr	tr	1	—
Squeeze	1 tsp	34	tr	tr	tr	3	—
Stick	1 tsp	34	0	tr	tr	1	—
MARSHMALLOW							
Marshmallow	1 reg (0.3 oz)	23	tr	0	0	0	tr
MATZO							
Plain	1 (1 oz)	112	3	0	4	4	1
Whole Wheat	1 (1 oz)	99	4	0	10	7	1
MILK							
1%	1 cup	102	8	2	12	300	tr
2%	1 cup	121	8	2	12	297	tr
Chocolate	1 cup	208	8	2	12	280	1
Condensed Sweetened	1 cup	982	24	8	34	868	1
Evaporated	1/2 cup	169	9	2	10	329	tr
Evaporated Skim	1/2 cup	99	10	2	11	369	tr
Goat	1 cup	168	9	3	1	326	tr
Nonfat	1 cup	86.	8	2	13	302	tr
Whole	1 cup	150	8	2	12	291	tr
MILK SUBSTITUTES							
Edensoy Carob	8 fl oz	150	6	0	38	67	2
Edensoy Original	8 oz	130	10	0	40	80	1

Food	Portion	Calories	Protein	Vit C	Folic Acid	Calcium	Iron
MILKSHAKE							
Thick Shake Chocolate	1 (16 oz)	719	18	5	9	631	3
Thick Shake Vanilla	1 cup (16 oz)	657	17	5	9	603	tr
MILLET							
Cooked	1 cup (6.1 oz)	207	6	0	33	5	1
MOLASSES							
Molasses	1 tbsp (0.7 oz)	53	0	—	0	41	1
MUFFIN							
Blueberry	1 (2 oz)	165	6	1	7	107	1
Bran	1 (2 oz)	164	4	5	30	106	2
Corn	1 (2 oz)	183	4	tr	10	147	1
MUSHROOMS							
Pieces	1/2 cup	19	1	—	10	—	1
Whole	1 (0.4 oz)	3	tr	—	2	—	tr
NECTARINE							
Fresh	1	67	1	7	5	6	tr
NOODLES							
Chow Mein	1 cup (1.6 oz)	237	4	0	39	9	2
Egg Cooked	1 cup (5.6 oz)	213	8	0	102	19	3
Lipton Noodles & Sauce							
Butter as prep	1 cup (2.2 oz)	310	8	0	100	0	3
Noodle Pudding	1/2 cup	132	6	1	8	51	1

Food	Portion	Calories	Protein	Vit C	Folic Acid	Calcium	Iron
Rice Cooked	1 cup (6.2 oz)	192	2	0	5	7	tr
OKRA							
Sliced Cooked	8 pods	27	2	14	39	54	tr
OLIVES							
Ripe	1 sm	4	tr	0	0	3	tr
ONION							
Chopped Cooked	1/2 cup	47	1	6	16	23	tr
Rings	2 (0.7 oz)	81	1	tr	3	6	tr
ORANGE							
Juice	1 cup	110	2	82	45	24	tr
Navel	1	65	1	80	47	56	tr
Sections	1 cup	85	2	96	55	52	tr
Tropicana Juice w/Calcium	8 fl oz	110	2	108	60	350	0
OYSTERS							
Battered & Fried	6 (4.9 oz)	368	13	4	13	27	4
Cooked	6 med	58	6	—	8	38	6
Stew	1 cup	278	15	4	14	331	6
PANCAKE/WAFFLE SYRUP							
Low Calorie	1 tbsp	12	0	0	0	—	—
Maple	1 tbsp (0.8 oz)	52	0	0	0	13	tr
Pancake Syrup	1 tbsp (0.7 oz)	57	0	0	0	0	tr

Food	Portion	Calories	Protein	Vit C	Folic Acid	Calcium	Iron
PANCAKES							
Potato	1 (4 in diam)	78	2	4	7	10	tr
W/Butter & Syrup	2 (8.1 oz)	520	8	4	30	128	3
PAPAYA JUICE							
Nectar	1 cup	142	tr	8	5	24	1
PARSNIPS							
Fresh Cooked	1/2 cup	63	1	10	45	29	tr
PASTA							
Elbows Cooked	1 cup (4.9 oz)	197	7	0	98	10	2
Lasagna	1 piece (2.5 in x 2.5 in)	374	22	13	11	359	3
Light Cheese Ravioli	1 cup	280	15	0	60	250	2
Macaroni & Cheese	1/2 cup	317	15	1	19	343	1
Manicotti	3/4 cup (6.4 oz)	273	14	12	17	76	3
Rigatoni w/Sausage Sauce	3/4 cup	260	10	16	8	44	3
Spaghetti Cooked	1 cup (4.9 oz)	197	7	0	98	10	2
Spaghetti w/Meatballs & Cheese	1 cup	407	21	45	22	164	5
Vegetable Pasta Cooked	1 cup (4.7 oz)	172	6	0	87	15	1
Whole Wheat Cooked	1 cup (4.9 oz)	174	7	0	7	21	1
PEACH							
Fresh	1	37	1	6	3	5	tr

Food	Portion	Calories	Protein	Vit C	Folic Acid	Calcium	Iron
Halves In Light Syrup	1 half	44	tr	2	3	3	tr
PEANUT BUTTER							
Chunky	2 tbsp	188	8	0	29	13	1
Jif Reduced Fat	2 tbsp (1.3 oz)	190	8	—	24	—	1
Skippy Reduced Fat	2 tbsp	190	9	0	24	0	1
Creamy Smooth	2 tbsp	188	8	0	25	11	1
PEANUTS							
Chocolate Coated	10 (1.4 oz)	208	5	0	3	42	1
Dry Roasted	1 oz	164	7	0	41	15	1
Mixed Nuts Salted	1 oz	169	5	tr	14	20	1
Planters Reduced Fat Honey Roasted	1/3 cup (1 oz)	130	6	0	60	20	1
PEAR							
Fresh	1	98	1	7	12	19	tr
Halves In Light Syrup	1 half	45	tr	1	1	4	tr
PEAS							
Green Cooked	1/2 cup	67	4	11	51	22	1
Green Raw	1/2 cup	58	4	29	47	18	1
PECANS							
Dry Roasted	1 oz	187	2	—	12	10	1
PEPPERS							
Green	1 (2.6 oz)	20	1	95	16	7	tr

Food	Portion	Calories	Protein	Vit C	Folic Acid	Calcium	Iron
Jalapeno	1 (0.5 oz)	4	tr	6	7	1	tr
Red	1 (2.6 oz)	20	1	141	16	7	tr
Yellow	10 strips	14	1	95	14	6	—
PERSIMMONS							
Fresh	1	118	1	13	13	13	tr
PICKLES							
Dill	1 (2.3 oz)	12	tr	1	1	6	tr
Sweet	1 (1.2 oz)	41	tr	tr	0	1	tr
PIE							
Apple	1/8 of 9 in pie (5.4 oz)	411	4	3	7	11	2
Blueberry	1/8 of 9 in pie (5.2 oz)	360	4	1	7	10	2
Cherry	1/8 of 9 in pie (6.3 oz)	486	5	2	12	18	3
Lemon Meringue	1/8 of 9 in pie (4.5 oz)	362	5	4	11	15	1
Pecan	1/6 of 8 in pie (4 oz)	452	5	1	7	19	1
Pumpkin	1/6 of 8 in pie (3.8 oz)	229	4	—	17	66	1

Food	Portion	Calories	Protein	Vit C	Folic Acid	Calcium	Iron
PIEROGI							
Pierogi	3/4 cup (4.4 oz)	307	11	1	8	156	2
PIKE							
Cooked	3 oz	96	21	—	3	62	1
PINEAPPLE							
Fresh Slice	1 slice	42	tr	13	9	6	tr
Juice	1 cup	139	1	27	58	42	1
Slices In Light Syrup	1 slice	30	tr	4	3	8	tr
PINK BEANS							
Cooked	1 cup	252	15	0	284	88	4
PINTO BEANS							
Cooked	1 cup	186	11	2	145	89	4
PISTACHIOS							
Dried	1 oz	164	6	—	17	38	2
PIZZA							
Cheese	1/8 of 12 in pie	140	8	1	59	116	1
Pepperoni	1/8 of 12 in pie	181	10	2	53	65	1
PLANTAINS							
Sliced Cooked	1/2 cup	89	1	8	20	2	tr
PLUMS							
Fresh	1	36	1	6	1	2	tr
Purple In Light Syrup	3	83	tr	1	3	13	1

Food	Portion	Calories	Protein	Vit C	Folic Acid	Calcium	Iron
POPCORN							
Air Popped	1 cup (0.3 oz)	31	1	0	2	1	tr
Mother's Popcorn Cake	1 (0.3 oz)	35	1	—	0	—	0
Oil Popped	1 cup (0.4 oz)	55	1	0	2	1	tr
POPOVER							
Popover	1 (1.4 oz)	90	4	tr	7	37	1
PORK							
Center Loin Roast	3 oz	169	23	1	3	21	1
Center Loin Chop Cooked	3 oz	172	25	1	3	20	1
Center Rib Chop Cooked	3 oz	213	23	tr	2	21	1
Chop Suey w/Pork	1 cup	375	19	58	24	36	3
Chow Mein Pork	1 cup	425	32	15	27	75	5
Fresh Ham Roasted	3 oz	232	23	tr	9	12	1
Ribs Country Style							
Braised	3 oz	252	20	1	3	25	1
Tenderloin Roasted	3 oz	139	24	tr	5	5	1
POTATO							
Baked Topped w/Cheese Sauce	1	475	15	26	28	310	3
Baked Topped w/Sour Cream & Chives	1	394	7	34	32	105	3
Baked w/Skin	1 (6.5 oz)	220	5	26	22	20	3

185

Food	Portion	Calories	Protein	Vit C	Folic Acid	Calcium	Iron
Boiled	1/2 cup	68	1	10	8	4	tr
French Fries	10 strips	111	2	6	8	4	1
Hash Brown	1/2 cup (2.5 oz)	151	2	6	8	7	tr
Instant Mashed as prep	1/2 cup	118	2	10	8	52	tr
Potato Puffs	1/2 cup	138	2	4	10	19	1
Potato Salad	1/2 cup	179	3	13	8	24	1
PRETZELS							
Chocolate Covered	1 (0.4 oz)	50	1	tr	—	8	tr
Sticks	60 (1 oz)	114	3	0	—	11	2
Whole Wheat	2 sm (1 oz)	103	3	0	—	8	1
PRUNE							
Dried	2	100	1	2	2	22	1
Juice	1 cup	181	2	11	1	30	3
PUDDING							
Bread Pudding	1/2 cup (4.4 oz)	212	7	1	16	143	1
Rice w/Raisins	1/2 cup	246	7	1	21	125	2
Snack Pack Chocolate	1 pkg (5 oz)	189	4	3	4	128	1
Snack Pack Vanilla	1 pkg (4 oz)	146	3	0	0	99	tr
Tapioca	1/2 cup (5.3 oz)	189	7	1	14	159	tr
RADICCHIO							
Raw Shredded	1/2 cup	5	tr	2	12	4	—

Food	Portion	Calories	Protein	Vit C	Folic Acid	Calcium	Iron
RADISHES							
Red Raw	10	7	tr	10	12	9	tr
RAISINS							
Seedless	1 cup	434	5	5	5	71	3
RASPBERRIES							
Frozen Sweetened	1 cup	256	2	41	65	38	2
RED BEANS							
Canned	1/2 cup (4.6 oz)	90	6	—	100	20	2
RICE							
Brown Cooked	1 cup (6.8 oz)	216	5	0	8	20	1
Cake	1 (0.3 oz)	35	1	0	2	1	tr
Glutinous Cooked	1 cup (6.1 oz)	169	4	0	2	3	tr
Instant Cooked	1 cup (5.8 oz)	162	3	0	68	13	1
Pilaf	1/2 cup	84	4	15	24	21	1
Spanish	3/4 cup	363	11	26	14	22	2
ROLL							
Brown & Serve	1 (1 oz)	85	2	—	8	34	1
Cinnamon Roll							
w/ Icing	1	686	62	1	75	50	2
Hard	1 (3 1/2 in)	167	6	0	8	54	2
Whole Wheat	1 (1 oz)	75	3	0	8	30	1

Food	Portion	Calories	Protein	Vit C	Folic Acid	Calcium	Iron
RUTABAGA							
Cooked Mashed	1/2 cup	41	1	26	19	50	1
SALAD							
Carrot & Raisin Salad	1 serv (4.5 oz)	321	2	11	1	41	1
Coleslaw	1/2 cup	42	1	20	16	27	tr
Tossed w/o Dressing	1 1/2 cups	32	3	48	77	26	1
Tossed w/o Dressing w/ Chicken	1 1/2 cups	105	17	17	67	37	1
Tossed w/o Dressing w/ Pasta & Seafood	1 1/2 cups (14.6 oz)	380	16	38	100	73	3
Waldorf	1/2 cup	79	1	2	6	12	tr
SALAD DRESSING							
French Reduced Calorie	2 tbsp	44	0	—	—	4	tr
Kraft Blue Cheese Free	2 tbsp (1 oz)	45	0	0	0	0	0
Newman's Own Oil & Vinegar	2 tbsp (1 oz)	150	0	0	0	0	0
Wishbone Chunky Blue Cheese	2 tbsp (1 oz)	150	1	0	0	20	0
SALMON							
Cake	1 (3 oz)	241	18	tr	7	203	1
Canned	3 oz	118	17	0	13	181	1
Lox (smoked)	1 oz	33	5	—	1	3	tr

Food	Portion	Calories	Protein	Vit C	Folic Acid	Calcium	Iron
SANDWICH							
Chicken Fillet w/ Cheese Lettuce Mayonnaise & Tomato	1	632	29	3	46	258	4
Fish Fillet w/ Tartar Sauce	1	431	17	3	44	84	3
Ham w/ Cheese	1	353	21	3	71	130	3
Roast Beef Plain	1	346	22	2	40	54	4
Roast Beef w/ Cheese	1	402	32	0	41	183	5
Steak w/ Tomato Lettuce Salt & Mayonnaise	1	459	30	6	89	91	5
Tuna Salad Submarine Sandwich w/ Lettuce & Oil	1	584	30	4	58	74	3
SARDINES							
Canned In Oil w/ Bone	2	50	6	—	3	92	1
Canned In Tomato Sauce w/ Bone	1	68	6	tr	9	91	1
SAUSAGE							
Breakfast	1 link (1/2 oz)	48	3	0	0	4	tr
SCALLOP							
Breaded & Fried	6 (5 oz)	386	16	0	40	18	2
SHERBET							
Orange	1/2 cup (4 fl oz)	132	1	4	4	52	tr

Food	Portion	Calories	Protein	Vit C	Folic Acid	Calcium	Iron
SHRIMP							
Breaded & Fried	6 to 8 (6 oz)	454	19	0	48	84	3
Chow Mein Shrimp	1 cup	221	13	15	28	105	3
Cooked	4 large	22	5	—	1	9	1
Jambalaya	3/4 cup	188	11	19	15	67	3
SODA							
Club	12 oz	0	0	0	0	17	—
Cola	12 oz	151	tr	0	0	9	tr
Diet Cola	12 oz	2	tr	0	0	12	tr
Ginger Ale	12 oz can	124	tr	0	0	12	tr
Orange	12 oz	177	0	0	0	19	tr
Root Beer	12 oz	152	tr	0	0	19	tr
SOLE							
Breaded & Fried	3.2 oz	211	13	0	51	17	2
SOUP							
Chicken Gumbo	1 serv (8 oz)	92	9	6	12	22	1
Chicken Noodle	1 cup	75	4	tr	2	17	1
Chicken Rice	1 cup	251	4	tr	1	17	1
Corn & Cheese Chowder	3/4 cup	215	9	7	12	220	1
Hot & Sour	1 serv (14 oz)	173	15	1	9	50	1
Onion Soup Gratinee	1 serv	492	25	11	57	637	2
Pasta E Fagioll	1 cup (8.8 oz)	194	9	12	49	62	3

Food	Portion	Calories	Protein	Vit C	Folic Acid	Calcium	Iron
Seafood Gumbo	1 serv (8 oz)	98	10	15	12	42	1
Split Pea w/ Ham	1 cup	189	10	1	3	22	2
Tomato	1 cup	86	2	67	15	13	2
Wonton	1 cup	205	16	5	15	32	3
SOUR CREAM							
Sour Cream	1 tbsp (0.4 oz)	26	tr	tr	1	14	tr
Substitute Nondairy	1 oz	59	1	0	0	1	—
SOY							
Soy Milk	1 cup	79	7	0	4	10	1
Soybeans Roasted & Toasted	1 cup	490	40	2	244	149	5
SPAGHETTI SAUCE							
Alfredo	1/4 cup (2.2 oz)	180	3	0	0	80	0
Alfredo Light	1/4 cup (2.4 oz)	140	5	0	0	100	0
Basil Pesto	1/4 cup (2.2 oz)	320	7	0	8	250	tr
Marinara	1/2 cup (4.5 oz)	70	2	0	0	40	1
SPANISH FOOD							
Burrito w/Beans & Cheese	2 (6.5 oz)	377	15	2	81	214	2
Chimichanga w/Beef	1 (6.1 oz)	425	20	5	31	63	5
Chimichanga w/ Beef & Cheese	1 (6.4 oz)	443	20	3	34	238	4

Food	Portion	Calories	Protein	Vit C	Folic Acid	Calcium	Iron
Enchilada w/ Cheese	1 (5.7 oz)	320	10	tr	34	324	1
Frijoles w/ Cheese	1 cup (5.9 oz)	226	11	2	111	188	2
Nachos w/ Cheese	6 to 8 (4 oz)	345	9	1	10	272	1
Taco	1 sm (6 oz)	370	21	2	23	221	2
Taco Salad	1 1/2 cups	279	13	4	40	192	2
Tamales	2 (5.1 oz)	210	6	–	8	20	1
Tostada w/Beans & Cheese	1 (5.1 oz)	223	10	1	75	211	2
Tostada w/Guacamole	2 (9.2 oz)	360	12	4	110	424	2
SPINACH							
Cooked	1/2 cup	21	3	9	131	122	3
Raw Chopped	1/2 cup	6	1	8	54	28	1
Spinach Tossed Salad	1 serv (4 oz)	88	3	14	72	103	1
STRAWBERRIES							
Fresh	1 cup	45	1	85	26	21	1
STUFFING/DRESSING							
Bread	1/2 cup	178	3	—	17	32	1
Stove Top Flexible Serve Homestyle Herb as prep	1/2 cup (3.3 oz)	170	3	0	16	20	1
SUGAR							
Maple	1 piece (1 oz)	100	0	0	0	26	tr
White	1 tsp (4 g)	15	0	0	0	0	0

Food	Portion	Calories	Protein	Vit C	Folic Acid	Calcium	Iron
SUNFLOWER							
Seeds Salted	1 oz	175	6	tr	67	16	2
SWEET POTATO							
Baked w/ Skin	1 (3 1/2 oz)	118	2	28	26	32	1
Candied	3 1/2 oz	144	1	7	12	27	1
TANGERINE							
Fresh	1	37	1	26	17	12	tr
Fresh Samantha Juice	1 cup (8 oz)	106	2	66	8	40	tr
TEA							
Brewed	6 oz	2	0	0	9	0	tr
TOMATO							
Fresh	1 (4.5 oz)	26	1	24	18	6	1
Juice	6 oz	32	1	33	36	16	1
Stewed	1 cup	80	2	18	11	27	1
TORTILLA							
Corn	1 (6 in diam)	56	1	0	4	44	tr
Flour	1, 8 in diam (1.2 oz)	114	3	0	4	44	1
TROUT							
Baked	3 oz	162	23	tr	13	47	2
TUNA							
Canned In Oil	3 oz	169	25	—	5	11	1

Food	Portion	Calories	Protein	Vit C	Folic Acid	Calcium	Iron
Canned In Water	3 oz	99	22	0	3	10	1
Tuna Salad	1 cup	383	33	5	15	35	2
TURKEY							
Breast w/ Skin Roasted	4 oz	212	32	0	7	24	2
Ground Cooked	3 oz	188	20	0	5	21	2
Leg w/ Skin Roasted	1 (1.2 lbs)	1133	152	0	49	176	13
Wing w/ Skin Roasted	1 (6.5 oz)	426	51	0	10	44	3
TURNIPS							
Cooked Mashed	1/2 cup (4.2 oz)	47	2	23	19	58	1
Greens Cooked	1/2 cup	15	1	20	85	99	1
VEAL							
Cutlet Braised	3 oz	172	31	—	15	7	1
Loin Chop Braised	1 chop (2.8 oz)	227	24	—	11	22	1
Parmigiana	4.2 oz	279	22	15	11	137	3
Sirloin w/ Bone Roasted	3 oz	171	21	—	13	11	1
VEGETABLES MIXED							
Mixed	1/2 cup	54	3	3	17	22	1
Peas & Carrots	1/2 cup	38	3	7	21	18	1
WAFFLES							
Plain	1, 4 in sq (1.2 oz)	88	2	0	17	77	1
WALNUTS							
English Dried	1 oz	182	4	1	19	27	1

Food	Portion	Calories	Protein	Vit C	Folic Acid	Calcium	Iron
WATERMELON							
Seeds Dried	1 oz	158	8	—	16	15	2
Wedge	1/16	152	3	47	10	38	1
WHEAT GERM							
Kretschmer Original	1/4 cup	103	9	0	106	14	0
WHIPPED TOPPINGS							
Cool Whip Original	2 tbsp (0.3 oz)	25	0	—	0	0	0
Nondairy Pressurized	1 tbsp (4 g)	11	tr	0	0	tr	tr
WHITE BEANS							
Canned	1 cup	306	19	0	171	191	8
WHITEFISH							
Smoked	1 oz	39	7	—	2	5	tr
WHITING							
Cooked	3 oz	98	20	—	13	53	tr
WILD RICE							
Cooked	1 cup (5.7 oz)	166	7	0	43	5	1
YOGURT							
Fruit Lowfat	8 oz	225	9	1	19	314	tr
Plain	8 oz	139	8	1	17	274	tr
Plain Lowfat	8 oz	144	12	2	25	415	tr
Plain No Fat	8 oz	127	13	2	28	452	tr
Vanilla Lowfat	8 oz	194	11	2	24	389	tr

Food	Portion	Calories	Protein	Vit C	Folic Acid	Calcium	Iron
YOGURT FROZEN							
Chocolate Soft Serve	1/2 cup (4 fl oz)	115	3	tr	8	106	—
Vanilla Soft Serve	1/2 cup (4 fl oz)	114	3	1	4	103	tr
ZUCCHINI							
Cooked	1/2 cup	14	1	4	15	12	tr

INDEX